MAD WOMAN

Also by Bryony Gordon:

The Wrong Knickers: A Decade of Chaos
Mad Girl
Eat, Drink, Run
Glorious Rock Bottom
No Such Thing As Normal

For young adults:

You Got This
Let Down Your Hair

BRYONY GORDON

MAD WOMAN

How to survive a world that thinks you're the problem

HEADLINE

Copyright © Bryony Gordon 2024

The right of Bryony Gordon to be identified as the Author of
the Work has been asserted by her in accordance with the
Copyright, Designs and Patents Act 1988.

First published in 2024 by
HEADLINE PUBLISHING GROUP

3

Dialogue on page 167 a reference from *Labyrinth* (1986).

Cataloguing in Publication Data is available from the British Library

Hardback ISBN 978 1 0354 0868 9
Trade paperback ISBN 978 1 0354 0869 6

Typeset in Berling by CC Book Production

Printed and bound in Great Britain by Clays Ltd, Elcograf S.p.A.

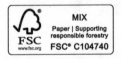

Headline's policy is to use papers that are natural, renewable and recyclable products
and made from wood grown in well-managed forests and other controlled sources.
The logging and manufacturing processes are expected to conform to the
environmental regulations of the country of origin.

HEADLINE PUBLISHING GROUP
An Hachette UK Company
Carmelite House
50 Victoria Embankment
London EC4Y 0DZ

www.headline.co.uk
www.hachette.co.uk

For all the younger versions of me,
and all the younger versions of you.

Contents

1

Never been better, thanks for asking

Snapshot from my iPhone's Notes App, December 2019

< Notes

Things I wood like when you go shopping. From Edie, age six-and-three-quarters.

peenutbuter

siryol

brokelee

food for my giny pig

my bedtime is 7 o colic can it be 8 o colic from edie

❮ Notes   ⬆️ ⋯

NY Resolutions for 2020

Travel more – explore world with Harry and Edie

Stop spending money on Deliveroo

Eat more brokelee

Have nice 40th birthday party

Find out more about e.g. Wim hof??

Smoke fewer cigarettes or even NONE

GET OUT OF YOUR OWN WAY

Save money? lol

Become the kind of person who reads Rumi, or even knows who Rumi is.

Oh ffs, stop having resolutions. Do you need to be better? You've done enough improving for the time being. Let the next ten years be a chance to REVEL IN YOUR AMAZINGNESS (eek!).

       ☑️   📷   Ⓐ   ✍️

It is the last day of the second decade of the twenty-first century, and I have never been happier. *Me*, Bryony Gordon, self-confessed alcoholic, professional fuck-up, dunderheaded depressive, recently described in a magazine as 'a poster girl for mental illness' ('Why couldn't you be a poster girl for Missoni instead?' asked my friend Holly, not unreasonably. 'That sounds like much more fun.') And despite all of this – *because* of all of this, perhaps – I am on cloud nine, or, more accurately, a beach in Phuket, sitting by a pool, staring out at the Andaman Sea, ten days into a two-week holiday with my husband and six-year-old daughter, about to see in the new year and the new decade in the most heavenly place possible.

Which is a bit of a turn-up for the books, isn't it?

On one side, my husband dozes on his sun lounger, sated after a lunch of tuna tartare and ice-cold Singha beer. On the other, my daughter plays in the shade with a selection of LOL Dolls she received a few days earlier for Christmas. The dolls are no bigger than the palm of her teeny-tiny hand, and yet still they manage to have freakishly big eyes and extravagantly coiffed hair. They are like Barbara Cartland in doll form. My child holds a tiny Barbara Cartland in each hand, lost in her own world of make-believe.

'I love your dress,' one doll says to the other in a squeaky voice.

'Thank you,' says the doll with the good dress. 'Your hair is fantastic. But do you know what is most important?'

'What's that?' replies the doll with the good hair.

'What's important is that *we* are fantastic! It doesn't matter how cool our outsides are. What matters is what is *inside* us!'

'Nothing but empty air in a hollow plastic shell,' mutters my husband under his breath, but luckily my daughter is too immersed in the world of her new Barbara Cartland friends to hear.

'Well, *I* think, on this day of all days, we should be grateful that this decade has given us a wonderful daughter who cares about what's on the inside of her LOL Dolls rather than the outside. Which is just as well, given that I think one of them is wearing' – I pick up a mini Barbara Cartland and squint at it in the light of the sun – '*fishnets.*'

'I do wish you'd stop going on about it being New Year,' grouches my husband. 'Not to mention the inappropriateness of children's toys nowadays. It makes me feel old.'

'We *are* old, Harry!' I am waving the fishnet-clad doll around in the air. 'And that's a good thing. Lots of people don't get to be old! And as for me going on about it being New Year's Eve – well, it's not as if it's just any New Year's Eve. It's the last day of the maddest decade we've ever experienced. Parenthood, marriage, house ownership . . .'

'God, you're making us sound exciting.'

'Rehab, books, podcasts, marathons, meeting Hugh Jackman on the plane . . .'

'These are all things you did.' Harry sighs.

'I couldn't have done them without you!' I am jazz-handing so hard that the fishnet-clad doll flies out of my hand, landing under the nearby sun lounger of a snoring tourist.

'Oh, come on now,' Harry says, raising his eyebrows. 'We both know New Year's Eve is just another silly excuse for people to stay up late and have a party. And you don't even *like* to stay up late and have a party anymore. Do we have to turn *everything* into a moment for deep reflection? I mean, time is just an abstract construct. Speaking of which, it's time for me to go and have a swim.'

Holiday shopping list of smug

- Face SPF as recommended by an Instagram influencer that is so expensive you only use it sparingly, thus ending up with sunburn.
- Beach bag that looks a bit like that Christian Dior one all the celebrities have but isn't actually the Christian Dior one all the celebrities have, because though you're feeling smug, you're not so smug that you are prepared to spend £2,500 on a bag that will get covered in sand and the Boots Soltan you should have put on your face instead of that stupid expensive Instagram SPF.

- Five-hundred-page novel that has been shortlisted for the Booker Prize, which you won't actually read but *will* position nonchalantly on your sun lounger when posing for holiday snaps to upload to social media.
- Sunglasses from Duty Free that will break on the second day of the trip when your husband flings them into the fake Christian Dior beach bag, where they will be crushed under the weight of the five-hundred-page book you won't get round to reading.

Harry gets up, blows me a kiss, and dives into the pool. I watch his shadow under the water, tracking it until he breaks the surface and starts waving at Edie, who has put down the remaining baby Barbara Cartland and is now making her way to join him. I admire my husband's blithe relationship with time, the fact he doesn't see it as anything other than a social construct to stop him being late. But for me, it is much more than that. Today may be 'just another' New Year's Eve to my husband, but to me, it is 856 days since I last had an alcoholic drink or a line of cocaine. What's more, it is two years, two months and sixteen days since my last OCD episode. It is 115 weeks since Jareth the Goblin King last sat in my frontal lobe, telling me I might be a serial-killing paedophile. It is 19,320 hours since I last worried my daughter might be taken away. It's 1,159,200 minutes since I last considered killing myself. And it is 69,552,000 seconds since I let go of a lifetime's belief that I am bad.

That is not meaningless. That is not nothing. That is not some fantasy I have created; it is real and tangible, and it reminds me of how very far I have come.

I was never very good at maths, but I realise now that numbers help me to make sense of things. They are perhaps the *only* thing that helps me to make sense of things. I think back to the turn of the last decade, ten years ago, and how much has changed. Ten years ago, I wanted to marry a man who already had a wife, a man whose only interest in me lay between my legs. Ten years ago, the most significant relationship in my life was actually with Jareth the Goblin King, an entirely fictional character I had decided was living inside my head (how's that for nuts?). Ten years ago, I was being held together by pay-day loans and bags of Quavers crisps. Ten years ago, I thought it was perfectly fucking normal to turn up two hours late to work carrying a steam iron in a Tesco carrier bag because I had spent all morning obsessively checking that it was off so that the flat didn't burn down, and in the end turning up to the office with my iron just felt like the easiest, most common sense thing to do.

Ten years ago, my default setting was worry. It was stress. It was despair. It was levels of anxiety so high that I didn't know it was unusual to go to bed every night scared you were going to die, or to wake up every morning somehow conversely wishing you had. Ten years ago, I thought recovery was something you did after a two-day cocaine bender. Ten years ago, ten years ago, ten years ago . . .

I am snapped out of my grim reverie by a shriek of delight from my daughter, who is enjoying being thrown repeatedly into the pool by my grinning husband.

And I sit and I catch myself and I look around at what I have now. There are the big things: the happy family, the sober life, the ability to wake up in the morning not absolutely filled with self-loathing. But then there are the smaller ones, which mean almost as much. The fact I am wearing a bikini made from recycled fishing nets that cost almost £150. The fact that when I post a picture of me in said bikini on Instagram, I get thousands of likes, because there is nothing the internet likes more than a woman over a size sixteen living her best life. The fact that – goddammit! – I am even *wearing* a bikini, given that most of my adult life has been spent feeling too big, and not bulimic enough. The fact I have not purged any food for – oh, I cannot even remember now, it's been that long. The fact that I have a normal relationship with food, and my body. The fact that I am the kind of person who is reading *The Road Less Travelled* by M. Scott Peck and *actually* getting something from it. The fact that I am not sitting here, on the beach, with Jareth obsessively asking me if I am sure that my daughter is actually my husband's, if I am sure that she is not the product of an encounter I blanked out in drunken horror, and if I am sure that I am not ruining the lives of everyone around me simply by existing. The fact that I feel safe. That I am not having to chant tiny prayers to a God I don't believe in to make sure that everyone I love stays alive. The fact that I have not had to bring my phone with me from the room, because I don't need it next to me at all times to reassure me that I haven't missed any calls from the neighbours telling me the house has burned down in our absence. The fact that I can go away at all, that I am not paralysed with fear at the thought of setting foot on a plane, that I haven't spent any of this holiday worrying that I might have hurt an innocent child while passing the kids' club and then blanked it out in shock. These are small things, but as anyone who has ever done battle with OCD will know, they are not unimportant things. In fact, they are *everything*.

I have fought hard for all of them. I have battled for each and every one of them. The language of war does not seem overblown to me – it's just that the enemy I was fighting a war against was myself. The fact that I have managed to step back from this constant battle and into a world of peace and contentment is only thanks to the army alongside me, made up of people I met through writing *Mad Girl* and setting up Mental Health Mates. The 'We' – who I now know are everywhere – who email me and write to me and come up to me in the street, and even on the plane on the way here, and remind me that I am not mad – or that I am mad, but that this is OK, because I'm not *bad*.

'Excuse me,' interrupts the man who was previously sleeping on the nearby sun lounger. 'I think this is yours.' He hands me the fishnet-clad LOL Doll, shoots me a look of mild disdain, and then steps into the pool and makes his way to the swim-up bar for a cocktail.

I sit on the lounger and look at the tiny doll in her fishnets. I think she is one of those LOL Dolls that will cry if you hold her underwater for thirty seconds and then squeeze her stomach. She looks sad, as well she might. She reminds me a bit of myself, at the turn of this decade: all dressed up, hoping someone might love me, but essentially empty inside except for tears. I hold her to my chest, and watch my husband and daughter howling with laughter in the pool. On the horizon, the sun is dipping below the ocean for the last time in 2019. On the beach, some people are sticking up a huge banner bearing the numbers 2020. The new year is on its way: the new decade.

'We're safe now,' I whisper to the doll. 'It's going to be OK.' I feel a tear drop down my own cheek – a happy one. For the first time in my life, I am going into a new decade feeling hopeful and happy. Like nothing could possibly go wrong.

A selection of sad-looking toys I have felt a deep affinity with over the years

Cabbage Patch Kids

I often like to complain that I grew up with unrealistic beauty standards that were foisted on me by the impossible proportions of Barbie dolls. But this is slightly disingenuous, because as well as Barbie dolls, my childhood featured Cabbage Patch Kids, who were the doll equivalent of Miriam Margolyes to Barbie's Margot Robbie. Patriarchal conditioning being as terrible then as it is now, my friends and I rejected the dumpy, doughy Cabbage Patch Kids as soon as we were old enough to demand Barbie. But if I had my time again, I'd be team Cabbage Patch Kid all the way.

Teddy Ruxpin

An early animatronic toy that was essentially a cassette player shaped like a teddy bear. Teddy Ruxpin would half-heartedly move its mouth along to the music or story you had placed in its back (a tape deck). Teddy Ruxpin did not seem into it. Teddy Ruxpin was essentially every child at school assembly being made to chant the Lord's Prayer or sing the hymn 'Morning Has Broken'.

Boglin

Hideous rubber hand puppets that provided an early opportunity to have conversations with the highly critical voice inside my head.

11

Tamagotchi

Like most children in the seventies, eighties and nineties, barely being kept alive by its owners.

Glo Worm

A sad-looking worm that was actually a night light you could cling onto if you were scared of the dark. Its tragic-looking face stared back at you in the dead of night, as if to say, 'I know, I know, if a monster crawls out from under the bed and I'm all you've got, we're both completely fucked.'

Hungry Hungry Hippos

My spirit animal.

2

Fine

Snapshot from my iPhone's Notes App, January–February 2020

< Notes

Exciting things to look forward to this year

Going to Miami for work at Easter!

Running third Marathon in April!

New book coming out + getting to go on tour in May!

Fortieth birthday in July!

Three years sober in August! (Touch wood!)

All sorts of exciting things that require multiple exclamation marks!!!!

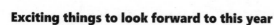

I'm fine.

Absolutely fine.

Fine and dandy. Fine like art, fine like wine, fine like ... fine.

'How are you today, Bryony?' I ask myself every morning, as I stare in the bathroom mirror.

'I'm fine, thank you so much for asking,' I reply, feeling really, perfectly fine.

Completely fine.

Fine, fine, *fine*.

I've spent the last few years of my career cautioning against too much use of the word 'fine', and yet, it's now the only one I appear to have in my vocabulary.

When I started my mental health podcast a few years ago, I decided the first question I would ask each of my guests was: 'How are you, *really?*'

'You're not allowed to say you're fine,' I snapped at the likes of Prince Harry, Stephen Fry and Sporty Spice, as if I was the kind of person who could tell the likes of Prince Harry, Stephen Fry and Sporty Spice what to do. '"Fine" is a cop-out word. It's a word you've got to watch for. It's a word that's employed when someone is absolutely *not* fine, but they're too polite or scared or ashamed to say otherwise.' Then I would make royalty – pop, television or literal – tell me their deepest, darkest feelings, and in the process we would do our tiny part to make the world at the very least *feel* like a better place.

It worked well, for a time.

But then ...

There's always a 'but then', isn't there?

But then ...

Well, you know what happened then.

*　　*　　*

A few weeks after we return from Thailand, my husband comes home from work and announces with complete certainty that we are on the brink of a pandemic, the likes of which has not been seen in our lifetimes. He says it as if he is telling me that his boss has been mildly annoying that day, or that there has been a ridiculous delay on the Northern Line that left him nestled in a stranger's armpit for twenty minutes.

'I think there's going to be a pandemic,' he says, taking off his suit jacket and sitting down on the sofa.

'That's nice,' I reply, hanging up wet washing to dry on the clothes horse. 'Do you think there's also going to be a time when we will get a tumble dryer? Because at the moment our home looks like a Victorian laundry.'

'I think this pandemic is more pressing than our need for a tumble dryer,' he shoots back, loosening his tie in that really annoying, passive-aggressive way men do, as if they are actually trying to say, 'I am MAN, I am IMPORTANT, I have BEEN OUT HUNTING ALL DAY FOR FOOD AND YOU SHOULD RESPECT ME!'

'Do you know what I think is really, truly the most pressing thing in our lives right now?' I turn to him, shaking out a sock stuck in a pair of leggings. 'It's that despite it being the year 2020, and me having a job that pays the majority of the mortgage, we still find ourselves slipping into these gendered stereotypes, whereby I find myself doing the washing while you stretch out on the sofa and tell me that there's going to be a pandemic, as if that's at all a constructive or helpful thing to say on a dark, gloomy, wet night in January. Now, come and help me hang these pants out to dry.'

He sighs, removes his tie completely, and picks up some knickers decorated with pictures of Olaf from *Frozen* (don't worry – not his).

'It's sweet that you're concerned there's going to be a pandemic.' I smile patronisingly. 'But I think you're being a wee bit overdramatic. I heard the Chinese have this virus totally under control. Which leaves us free to make a plan for that tumble dryer.'

'Bryony, I don't think—'

'Take it from me: I'm not worried about this. And I'm someone who spent my childhood washing my hands until they bled because I was so scared of germs. If, despite being a sufferer of Obsessive Compulsive Disorder, *I'm* not bothered about it, then you can chill your boots.'

'Chill your boots?' says Harry, completely mystified. 'What are you? Fifteen?'

'I think you'd be hard-pushed to find a fifteen-year old who would be caught dead saying "chill your boots".' I roll my eyes. 'I've seen a good Bosch on offer at Currys, by the way.'

'Seriously, Bryony, will you just listen to me? I think you *should* be worried.'

I stare at the miniature T-shirt in my hands, the one that says 'FOLLOW YOUR DREAMS'. I'm not sure how long I spend looking at the squiggly hearts and flowers on it, but it is long enough that when I finally look up, Harry has broken into a sweat.

'Did you just tell me to . . . worry?'

His face turns a little pale.

'We've known each other for, what, almost ten years now. And in that time, what would you say was your most-used phrase when talking to me?'

He shifts uncomfortably and picks up another pair of *Frozen* knickers.

'Would you agree,' I continue, 'that the thing you say most often to me is . . .'

18

I pause for dramatic effect.

He has now turned red.

'... "Don't worry"?'

'Well yes, that's probably the thing I've said most often to you.' He gulps.

'More so than even "I love you".'

'Now listen, Bryony, I think you're miss—'

'When I first got on a plane with you, and became convinced it was going to fall out of the sky, what did you say to me?'

'Don't worry,' he says, unable to look me in the eye.

'When I went through that period when OCD convinced me every day that I had sent a rude email to my boss and then deleted it in horror, what did you say to me?'

He clears his throat. 'Don't worry.'

'And when I couldn't leave the house because I was sure that I was a terrible person and everyone hated me, what did you say to me?'

'Don't worry?'

I nod. 'Furthermore, when I was pregnant with our daughter, and the OCD kept telling me that maybe our daughter wasn't actually yours and I had cheated on you and blanked it out in disgust, and I actually *told* you this, to seek some sort of twisted reassurance, what did you say to me?'

'I told you not to worry,' he says. 'And thanks for that reminder.'

'Would you say, having got to know me reasonably well by this point – this point being the fact we own a house together, have a child together and once even spent a day kayaking together without filing for divorce – that I am something of a worrier?'

'I mean, yes.' He sighs. 'That would be a fair description of you.'

'Would you say that I worry when I don't have anything to

worry about, and that I have done a fair amount of work on trying to make myself a less anxious person?'

'That would be a reasonable assessment, yes.'

'So after all of this time telling me not to worry about things, you are now informing me that I should *actively be worried* about something happening thousands of miles away in a fish market?'

'Kind of, yes. And actually, it's a wet market. It also sold meat.'

'My apologies. A wet market that sold meat as well as fish.' I glare at my husband.

'Look, darling, I appreciate you get anxious about things,' he says. 'And I'm not encouraging you to panic. I'm just saying that when the Chinese lock down an entire city and start disinfecting the streets, then it's probably a good idea to start preparing.'

'Preparing? What, like stocking up our bunker with canned food and putting on tin foil hats?'

He rolls his eyes. 'It's just what I'm hearing from my colleagues in Hong Kong.'

'It's just what I'm hearing from my colleagues in Hong Kong,' I parrot, in my most babyish voice.

'Don't say I didn't warn you.' He hangs up the last pair of *Frozen* pants on the drying rack.

'I won't say that, but only because in a couple of weeks' time, the world will have moved on and we will have completely for-gotten we ever had this conversation. Though hopefully not the bit about the tumble dryer. In the meantime, I would just like to reiterate, for the record, that I AM NOT WORRIED. Not in the slightest. Now, let me show you the Bosch.'

Worries I've had that haven't happened (yet)

- Monster under the bed coming and eating me and my Glo Worm.
- Falling off the ghost train and into a parallel universe where I have to battle dragons.
- Acid rain burning holes in everything, including my brain.
- A flood washing away London.
- An alien invasion.
- Drowning in a pool because I didn't wait half an hour after eating before I swam.
- Being sucked into quicksand.
- Teddy Ruxpin somehow turning into Chucky from *Child's Play*.
- Everyone hating me.
- Being the worst person in the world.
- My friend not replying to a WhatsApp because I did something terrible I can't actually remember.
- The plane I am in falling out of the sky.
- Being cancelled for something I tweeted while drunk/ high in 2007.
- Everything I love being taken away from me.

Worries I haven't had that *have* happened

- Donald Trump becoming president.
- Covid.

What does this tell you? Always worry.

When I was twelve years old, I woke up one morning convinced that I was dying of AIDS. I believed it with every beat of my heart, every breath that anxiously escaped from my lungs – each breath, I was convinced, one of my last. The night before, I had gone to bed a reasonably happy adolescent girl who had just been lucky enough to attend the *Smash Hits* Poll Winners Party (if you were born in the eighties, you'll know what I am talking about), the only hint of trouble being the fact that Robbie Williams had lost out to Mark Owen in the Most Fanciable Male category *again* (when would people realise Robbie was the greatest member of Take That? About ten years later, as it turns out, but I had yet to learn the valuable lesson that everybody blossoms in their own good time).

That night, I dreamed not of this injustice, but that I had an incurable illness. The dream felt hyper real, and in the morning, when I woke up, I became convinced that it was actually true. There was a voice in my brain telling me that I had AIDS, and that I was bad, and I knew I had to listen to it. If I didn't, I would end up infecting my family and killing them.

At the time, there was a terribly shaming 'public health' campaign about HIV and AIDS that really only served to stigmatise the gay community who were being so terribly affected by this pandemic. I can see that now, but I couldn't at the time. I was only twelve, and my brain was too juvenile to appreciate any awful truth other than the one being peddled by this strange, all-knowing voice in my frontal lobe.

'You probably have AIDS,' it said. 'You think you are healthy, but don't those adverts say that most people die of ignorance, that they don't find out they have it until it's too late? That's you. You're going to die of AIDS. And you are going to pass it to your family, including your newborn brother, and you will be responsible for them dying. You are a bad person. A terrible person. You are poison, you are deadly, you are shame.'

Everywhere I looked, I saw danger. Killer germs lurked on every surface. I would go to sleep with my toothbrush under my pillow, in fear that I might infect my sister. I was terrified of anything red, because it could hide blood. I began to wash my hands obsessively, before long hundreds of times a day, until my skin became so dry that it cracked and bled. This was another level of terror – suddenly, my hands felt like weapons, capable of infecting anyone they came near. I was too scared to wear gloves – what if they hid some other illness? – but was OK with pockets, because somehow they felt safer, perhaps more washable.

I've said this before and I will say it again and again and again: there was no logic to what was going on in my head – a rhyme, maybe, a never-ending death song, but absolutely no reason. Some people have music that gets stuck in their heads, but I had phrases that were caught on a loop, repeated endlessly in the hope that they would protect my family from this awful disease.

'I'd rather I died than my brother,' went round and round and round my brain, until I was whispering it under my breath in any spare moment that I wasn't washing my hands, as if it was some jaunty pop song. In time, I felt too scared to go out. I stayed in my room, my funny little quirks put down to moody adolescence. If you think mental health provision for children sucks now – and it does – you should see what was around in the nineties. Zilch. Zip. Nothing. Nada. I spent a few months in absolute terror, and then, just as quickly as the thoughts had come, they went away again.

I didn't think about them again until a few years later, when I was studying for my A levels. It was then that my fear about dying of AIDS returned, and it was then that I discovered the illness I had was not a physical one, but a mental one: Obsessive Compulsive Disorder (OCD). OCD is a debilitating condition that causes intrusive thoughts so uncontrollable that the sufferer engages in a series of compulsions to try and ease them. This, however, only feeds into the loop, and makes the intrusive thoughts worse. OCD is a convincing liar, telling you the most awful things about yourself until it becomes almost impossible to believe anything else is true. It's like living with Donald Trump, 24/7, with no ability to get away from him. In other words: hell.

And yet so often it is used as a jokey term that is code for being tidy. And I am not tidy. 'I wish you had the *good* type of OCD,' my husband often jokes now, at which point I have to lecture him on how there is no 'good' type of Obsessive Compulsive Disorder – the key word being *disorder*. But the point is, I am messy. So messy that my brain has often felt like it is going to explode, leaving even more mess on the kitchen counter. It's hard to describe OCD to people who think it exists only in their super-organised sock drawer, but I'll have a go. OCD, I have come to realise, is when your brain refuses to acknowledge what your eyes can see. It's when your brain won't believe that your hands are clean, that you couldn't possibly have HIV because you are a twelve-year-old girl who has never even kissed a boy and whose drug habit is at least a decade in the future. It's when your brain won't believe that the oven is switched off, that the iron is unplugged, that your family are safe and, furthermore, that chanting phrases to keep them alive will have absolutely no bearing on whether they live or die. It's when your brain throws violent, sometimes sexual thoughts into your consciousness, thoughts that make you feel sick, that make you want to die. It's when your brain tells you that those thoughts you have no control over, and that you would never act on, are a sign that you're evil. It's when your brain refuses to believe that you are a decent person who just happens to have a horrible mental illness.

Things OCD isn't:

- Having an organised sock drawer.
- Liking things to be tidy and neat.
- A passion for ironing.
- The odd, fleeting anxiety that you left the front door open.
- A hilarious and kooky quirk.

Things OCD is:

- A vicious, awful illness that involves hideous intrusive thoughts, exhausting compulsions, and quite often suicidal tendencies.

At some point, I called my OCD 'Jareth the Goblin King', after the character in the 1980s movie *Labyrinth* who was played by David Bowie. I remember, as a child, finding Jareth ever-so-slightly attractive (was it the tight silver trousers?) even though I knew he was bad. To me, that was how my OCD felt: evil, and yet maddeningly seductive.

Over the following decades – through several breakdowns, one agonising trip to rehab, and a hell of a lot of connection with people like you – I had learned to manage Jareth. It had become my life's work to help other people who might secretly have a Jareth living in their head. In doing so, I had got to the point where I could stand up on a stage in front of a thousand people and joke about Jareth. I had gone on national television and told Lorraine Kelly about Jareth. Jareth was no more than a slightly bothersome prick, and I had learned how to put him in his place – his place being the very, very back of my head, the bit where you store all those things that are no longer useful to you, like New Kids On The Block lyrics, your first boyfriend's landline number, that kind of thing.

So you'll understand when I tell you that my husband's pre-diction about this so-called pandemic leaves me behaving like a meerkat standing on its hind legs, frozen in place, completely still, preparing to make a dash from a poisonous snake that's ready to gobble it for breakfast.

Suddenly, I am on red alert, not necessarily because of the impending pandemic, but because he's given me a reason to think Jareth might creep forward in my head. Because, let's face it, a pandemic is exactly the kind of crazy-arse event that someone with OCD spends a disproportionate amount of time worrying about. It's exactly the kind of thing that I have been planning for since I was twelve. It's exactly the kind of thing I've been made to feel like an idiot for caring about. It's exactly the kind of ludicrous concern I have stored away in the back of my head, along with Jareth and the lyrics to every single song on the *Step by Step* album. And now, after a lifetime of being told I was overthinking things, or making a fuss about nothing, or being *overdramatic*, those same people are informing me that actually, I may have had a point.

What the . . .?

Conversations with my mother: Part one

'I told you the world was going to end,' I say to my mum one night on the phone, when she rings to tell me a rumour she's heard from Kelly who works in Waitrose, who heard it from Mike, her second cousin, who heard it from his mate Steve, who works in the civil service.

'They've started building secret underground graves to be able to handle all the dead bodies,' she whispers to me, presumably in case her dog overhears her.

'Who's "they", mum? Is it the SAS? Is it the Secret Service? The KGB?'

'The government!'

'Boris Johnson and Matt Hancock are building secret under-ground graves? Cor blimey! Still, I suppose it would be bad if they were planning to bury people *above* the ground.'

'I think you're being facetious,' snaps my mum.

'I think you're spreading panic,' I snap back. 'Which I could do without, given the fact that it's 8pm and I still haven't managed to get the child to sleep.'

'For someone who has spent most of their life worrying about this kind of thing, I have to say I am remarkably surprised that you don't seem to be taking this in the least bit seriously.'

'I have other things I need to take seriously, like the six-year-old insisting that she should be allowed to sleep in the guinea pig's hutch.'

'I imagined you'd be walking around spraying hand sanitiser at anyone who dared to cross your path.'

'Gotta go,' I say sweetly. 'Amazon have just turned up to deliver my Hazmat suit. Stay safe!'

I put the phone down and shake my head.

*   *   *

Am I in denial?

Why am I not scared of this virus at all, other than the potential it might have to wake up Jareth?

How selfish am I?

I go and see my therapist, Peter, who was my counsellor back in 2017, and whom I still check in with once a month. After all, when you're an alcoholic depressive with a history of eating disorders and OCD, it's important to have an anchor in your life.

Peter has seen me at my worst. And my worst is so bad that, at times, it makes Keith Richard's worst look like a best. He – Peter, not Keith Richard – knows my deepest, darkest secrets, ones I have not told anyone, not even as someone who is prone to writing about their deep darkness in books (would it surprise you if I told you that there's loads of stuff I haven't published? I mean, let's not get into that). Telling him I am a bit worried that I'm *not* worried about a pandemic feels quite minor in the grand scheme of things. Possibly a little ... self-indulgent?

'I'm a bit embarrassed about this,' I announce as soon as I sit down, 'but I feel like the whole point of you is to listen in a safe and non-judgemental way to things that embarrass me.'

Peter nods. I wonder if I've become more insufferable to him over the years, or less. We definitely have clearer boundaries now; when I first met him, and he told me that a boundary was a way of drawing a line around something, I asked him – jokingly, of course – if it was OK to then snort that line.

Reader, he didn't laugh.

But I haven't even thought about snorting lines of anything for a good couple of years. And as for my boundaries ... well, I've learned absolutely nothing about this man who knows absolutely everything about me, but what I do know is that this is a very important boundary for him. For example, I've realised that it's utterly pointless to ask him how he is, as he will just turn it back around to me, in that annoying way therapists have of not being easily distracted by mad clients who want to avoid talking about their madness at all costs (£100 a session, in case you were wondering).

'So the thing is, this virus everyone is talking about, I feel like Jareth should be all over it. A pandemic should be total catnip for him. Like Christmas for Mariah Carey, or Blue Monday for wellness brands seeking to make a quick buck out of your depression. And yet, he doesn't seem in the least bit interested in it. Try as I might – and I've been *really* vigilant about this – I can't find him. I can't say this to anyone else, but it would appear that I, despite surely being one of the world's most anxious people, am actually quite chilled about a killer disease that apparently seems certain to spread across the planet and change all of our lives forever.'

I think that just about sums it up.

'Right, and the fact you are clearly quite calm in the face of something quite frightening is a bad thing, how, exactly?'

'Well ...' I sit and ponder that one for a moment. 'I guess it's a bad thing because it means I'm a bad person. Like, if I cared about elderly and vulnerable people, I'd be way more concerned about this than I am. I would be freaking out. And I'm not. Which clearly means that Jareth's been right all along. I *am* wrong, and I *am* a freak, despite all this work I've done to try and prove otherwise.'

'I mean, that's one take. And it's a take that tells me that Jareth is actually alive and well, despite what you think. He may not be manifesting as a fear of germs, but maybe he's manifesting as the king of all OCD fears, which is the fear that you're a bad person. Instead of just accepting your reaction to what is happening, you're having to question it, and clearly quite rigorously. However you respond is the right response, because it's yours.'

I would call Peter a smart-arse if he wasn't a highly qualified professional with degrees coming out of his ears.

'But I clearly *am* a bad person, because if I was a good one, I would not be self-indulgently wanging on to you about this. I would be using this time to talk about my concerns for my mum living out in the country with only her dog and the occasionally mad theories of Kerry in Waitrose for company.'

'Bryony, I'm interested in this concept of what it means to be a bad person. Why you feel the need to split the world into bad and good. Surely it's healthier to accept we are all a mixture of everything?'

'So you're saying I *am* a bad human?'

He smiles. 'No, Bryony. I'm just saying that you're a human.'

We are standing in Sainsbury's on Clapham High Street, trying to buy toilet paper.

A few weeks ago, such an outing would not have warranted a mention in a text message, let alone a book.

But then . . .

Well, but then.

'There's no bog roll, Haz,' I say, stating the bleeding obvious.

'I can see that.'

'What are we going to do?' I keep looking at the empty shelves, as if the Andrex puppy might rush along one of them at any moment, pushing an unspooling roll of toilet paper that we might be able to claim for our home.

'Not go to the loo?'

'That's helpful.'

30

'I'm sorry, I'm trying to think.'

'Haven't your colleagues in Hong Kong got any advice on how to deal with toilet roll shortages?'

'Are you being sarcastic?'

'If you need to ask, Harry. If you need to ask.'

'I think the best thing is not to panic and try the Co-op.'

'Oh, *now* you don't want me to panic.'

Co-op is out.

There is a 750-metre queue to get into Tesco.

A security guard stationed at the entrance to Asda laughs when we ask if there's any loo roll in store.

We eventually procure some from a newsagent near Clapham Junction Station.

I am not just looking for loo roll. I am also looking for Jareth.

But, much like the bog roll, I can't find him anywhere.

Harry says that this is the first time he has seen me calmer than everyone else.

'Everyone's panicking, and you're behaving like a fucking Keep Calm and Carry On poster,' he mutters, when rumours start swirling about the country going into a lockdown similar to the ones already happening in Italy, Spain and France.

'I'm just not sure how much help it would be for me to have a breakdown right now,' I say, thinking that, actually, the look I was going for was 'shrugging emoji'.

'The timing of a breakdown has never bothered you before,' he says, not entirely unreasonably. For example, it wasn't ideal to have to go to rehab the day before our daughter started her first year at school, and I can't imagine it was particularly useful when I had a break from reality the day that he had to deliver a major project to his boss. Still, I resent the implication that I might be able to choose how crashingly depressed I feel on any given day, as if my mental state is a dress I pick out of a wardrobe of a morning. The only explanation I have for this apparent calm in the eye of the storm is that, as a person with a history of mental illness, I am used to panic. Because of the endless chaos that Jareth has caused inside my head over the years, I now find it quite easy to deal with chaos taking place outside of it. It's as if all those things that previously felt like flaws – OCD, addiction – have, in the face of a real pandemic, actually turned out to be strengths.

I spent all that time worrying that bad things might happen so that I wouldn't have to worry when they actually *did*.

'Maybe mental health issues are actually my superpower,' I mumble back to my husband, but he's scrolling through his phone, reading panicked tweets from sane people who have gone mad.

I am standing in the kitchen making our daughter dinner. My husband has been working from home for a week now, and I have not yet been able to vocalise how much I like it, both of us being here in the house, as if we are on some sort of weird working staycation. We eat lunch together, go for walks and hold hands. It is, objectively, really, really *nice*. But I feel that saying this out loud might somehow be treasonous. It would be insensitive, and the universe would pick up on my insensitivity and then punish me for it. So I say nothing. I go through the motions. I stop making jokes. Jokes feel like things from another time.

Instead of jokes, we now have daily Covid briefings. There is one on the radio now, as I do the egg-fried rice. The prime minister is talking about the need for certain groups of people to 'shield'. I am chopping spring onions, and he is saying that there is a possibility that vulnerable and elderly people will have to stay indoors for twelve weeks. Twelve whole weeks, inside, without seeing anyone at all.

I feel something spread through my body. It reminds me of what I felt when my daughter was two weeks old, and I went to the pub and got blackout drunk. It's a strange feeling, a kind of crawling sensation spreading through the skin that says, 'No, this can't be right. This isn't how things work. I am surely dreaming.'

Now, as back then, the sensation is followed by something leaking out of my eyes. Whatever it is drops on to the kitchen counter. I sniff and wipe it away. It keeps coming. The spell is finally broken by someone tapping me on the shoulder. I jump in shock, and see it is my husband.

'Did you hear the briefing?' he asks.

I turn away so he can't see me, and use a tea towel to wipe my eyes. If he asks, I will pretend it was the onions.

'I did.' I switch off the gas. 'I can't believe this is happening.' Before he can say anything, I cut across his path to reach for the cupboard containing the soy sauce. 'Can you tell Edie dinner is five minutes away and she needs to set the table?'

'Are you OK?' asks my husband, because as a newspaper journalist, it is not like me to shy away from a long and depressing conversation about Boris Johnson.

'Me?' I say, turning round and smiling as I wipe my hands on the tea towel. 'I'm fine!'

But even if I'm not fine, I'm hardly going to say so.

Not when, within weeks, the schools are shut and we are in lockdown, and I'm trying to make sure that my daughter still has a really, really great day turning seven.

Not when hundreds of people are dying every day.

Not when many more are lying prone in intensive care units, hooked up to ventilators.

Not when people are unable to see their gravely ill loved ones other than on the screen of an iPad, when the NHS staff, who are working round the clock at great risk to their own lives, can find a moment to help them FaceTime.

Not when all over social media, people are shaming the strangers they saw that day when taking their daily exercise. The strangers who have chosen to lie down on grass, sunbathing, when they know this is irresponsible. The strangers who have gone for a run and potentially let their sweat particles dispense all over good, upstanding citizens who are just trying to walk their dogs. The strangers who don't appear to understand what two metres entails, and who should be thoroughly ashamed of themselves because of this. The strangers who are directly responsible for the death of someone's granny because they selfishly left the house twice in one day. Shame on them. Shame on anyone who doesn't follow the rules. Shame, shame, shame.

So, I am fine.

Fine, fine, fine.

I am *fine*.

But I am finding that it is perfectly possible to be both fine and a little bit ashamed at the same time.

I am fine because I have a whole house and a small garden, and I am ashamed because I want to leave it more than once a day, while there are people out there living in one-bed flats with barely any space to swing a cat.

I am fine because I have a loving family, and I am ashamed because I am starting to find home-schooling annoying and my husband a pain, as if there aren't people out there with multiple children or no children at all, just an abusive relationship or a paralysing sense of loneliness.

I am fine because I have a job, and I am ashamed because I am struggling to juggle that job with home-schooling while there are people on furlough, or whose small businesses and livelihoods have been completely wrecked by Covid.

I am fine because . . .

Ooooh, is that you, Jareth?

'No!' says Jareth, slipping into a Boris Johnson mask, an ill-fitting suit, and a barely brushed blond wig. 'It is your Prime Minister, telling you to stay indoors and save lives and most of all, STOP BEING SELFISH! How can you be thinking about your mental health at a time like this, when people are dying and suffering, and you are privileged and healthy, and all I am asking you to do is sit at home on the sofa, watching Netflix? This is not the Second World War, Bryony. You are not being sent to the fucking trenches and forced to watch your friends being blown up by the Nazis. You know your great grandparents, who were driven out of their homes in the pogroms in Russia? THEY WOULD HAVE GIVEN ANYTHING TO SWAP THEIR CIRCUMSTANCES FOR A FEW WEEKS SITTING ON THEIR ARSES EATING BANANA BREAD AND WATCHING *ANT AND DEC'S SATURDAY NIGHT TAKEAWAY*! What bit of "this is not about you" do you fail to understand? Why are you so thoughtless? All you ever wang on about is mental health this, and mental health that, but let me tell you this, young lady. NOBODY CARES!'

I'm fine, you know. Just fine.

3

Chorizo

Snapshot from my iPhone's Notes App, April 2020

Sweaty Betty High Waisted Running Leggings Olive Leopard Print
Sweaty Betty High Waisted Running Leggings Black Tonal Scale Print
Sweaty Betty High Waisted Running Leggings Beetle Blue

But, if there is one teeny-tiny, absolutely *miniscule* way in which I am not fine, then it is probably evidenced in the raw cooking chorizo I have started eating in bulk, in secret, at two in the morning.

Very specifically, the Sainsbury's own-brand cooking chorizo.

None of that posh artisan stuff for me. Not when it costs as much as gold, and I'm eating as much of it as I am.

I tend to wash down a couple of packets of the raw cooking chorizo with a couple of packets of beef jerky. My husband has started buying the beef jerky because he says it is high in protein, which he needs thanks to the intensive exercise routine he has taken up to help him cope with the pandemic. As I inhale another packet of his beef jerky (not a euphemism), I wonder, when, exactly, I am going to become the kind of person who uses intensive exercise routines to cope with things. Not this lockdown, it would seem.

On top of this shame, I feel an extra added layer of shame about the type of food I can't stop eating. Some people go mad for Ben and Jerry's. Others can't resist a salt and vinegar crisp. But for me, only raw chorizo seems to hit the spot. Why couldn't it be raw broccoli, or raw carrots? Why coarsely chopped pork with paprika and garlic?

It's kind of *niche*.

There are a few things you can surmise from my strange eating habits. Firstly, that I am very much not fine. And secondly, that I would very much struggle to become a vegan, or a vegetarian, or even someone who just occasionally partakes in Meat-Free Monday.

What is it that happens to me, in those strange twilight-zone days of the first lockdown? Like many people, I am so busy trying to prove that I am fine, trying to find things for which I need to be grateful, that I clean forget to acknowledge that it would be perfectly ... well, *fine*, to be a bit freaked out by everything that has happened. I mean, one minute we were all singing 'Auld Lang Syne', getting excited for a new decade, and the next we were being locked down and told we could only leave the house once a day – or twice on Thursdays, when we would be allowed to step outside our front doors and clap for members of a health service buckling under the weight of a government that had failed to make any competent plans, or take any proper scientific advice. But it is not good to say these things. Saying these things might make me a bad person, and I don't want to feel like a bad person, because that's when Jareth pops up and starts wreaking havoc in my life. And at the moment – touch wood, oh please, God, let there be some wood near me, and if there isn't, will my head do? – Jareth is conspicuous only by his absence. So I tell myself everything is fine – just *fine!* – and I clap for carers and bake banana bread and home-school my child and hang rainbows in my window, along with signs that say things like 'HOPE'. I don't tell anyone that I dream of swimming in the sea, and seeing a skyline not dotted with concrete. I don't tell anyone that I yearn to be able to see versions of my friends that are not pixelated, that I fantasise about running away to Cornwall and taking the ferry across the River Fal to St Mawes, where we will get fish and chips and sit on the beach skimming stones into the sea.

I don't tell anyone these things, but I still feel them, and because I feel them, I know that deep down inside, I am a bad person.

I can sort of ignore my inherent badness during the day, because I am too busy to dwell on it. But in bed late at night, it starts to eat me alive. I toss and turn, unable to sleep as the badness sweeps through me, fizzing through every cell in my body. A few years ago, I would have gotten drunk on this feeling. I would have anaesthetised myself with booze. But I can't do that now, and so instead, I eat.

I creep downstairs, where the only light comes from the timer on the microwave. I kneel in front of the cupboard, find the jerky, and then make my way to the fridge, where I locate the packets of cooking chorizo where I have hidden them, deep at the bottom of the fruit and vegetable drawer that nobody ever looks in. I feel a swell of relief go through me as my fingers close around the plastic packet. Then I tiptoe into the living room, my bounty clutched to my chest, and in the dark, I eat. I eat and I eat and I eat, until there are threads of chorizo stuck in my teeth and my throat is dry from all the salt in the jerky and I feel suitably sedated. Then I put the wrappers in a plastic bag and hide them down the back of the sofa, from where I will retrieve them tomorrow, when nobody is looking, on my way out to replace Harry's beef jerky.

I am fine.

Late-night chats with my fridge

Me *(lying in bed, tossing and turning, unable to sleep)*: Why, oh why, does my brain insist on being slow, sluggish and semi-switched off during the day, only to come alive the moment my head hits the pillow?

Harry: *Snores.*

Me: I wish there was someone to talk to in these dark, lonely hours, but all I have is ...

Startles at beeping sound from downstairs, which I realize is the noise the fridge door makes when it has been left open too long.

Me: What the ...?

Harry: *Snores.*

Tentatively, I creep downstairs to the kitchen to investigate, and realise that the sound I can hear is coming from the fridge, it's door opening and closing as it, hang on, talks *to me.**

Fridge: Good evening, Bryony.

Me: What the fuck?

Fridge: Please don't swear; it offends the vegetables.

Me: The vegetables?

Fridge: The dairy and meat don't mind so much, and your husband's beers couldn't give a BLEEP BLEEP BLEEP, but the salad items are a little more sensitive.

Me: I think I'm losing it.

Fridge: I had noticed.

Me: What do you mean you'd noticed?

Fridge: Well, you've been dipping into me at strange times of the night. It's how we know our owners are stressed. So I thought I'd just check in and see how you were doing. We fridges like to call out to our owners when we sense they are in distress.

Me: You do?

Fridge: Yes. Usually in the dead of night, but not exclusively. The second most common time to call to an owner in distress is around 4pm, when you all tend to have the dreaded sugar crash, or at around 11am on a Saturday morning, when you come round from whatever you've been up to the night before. But to be fair, you don't tend to do that anymore. Which is a relief, because there was a point when my contents were eighty per cent alcohol, twenty per cent ready meals, and I considered staging an intervention. So many bits of me, not used for their proper purpose! The salad drawers filled with bottles of cava! The egg holder containing shots of ginger and turmeric, and those eye masks that were *not* going to balance out the amount of alcohol you were imbibing of an evening.

So I suppose this is an improvement. Of sorts.

Me: Are you policing my behaviour?

Fridge: I'd never be that strict. I'm pretty, you know, *chilled*.

Me: Very good.

Fridge: Anyway, I just wanted you to know that I'm always here for you in the dead of night when your husband is conked out snoring but your mind is racing and it feels like you are all alone. You can always count on me to soothe your tortured soul with some processed meat or cheese.

Kitchen cupboard: And if he's not able to help, there's always my nuts.

Me *(jumping out of my skin)*: You frightened me!

Kitchen cupboard: Sorry. Just wanted to let you know that I'm here for you too. Crisps. Beef Jerky. Cereal. All part of the service.

Fruit bowl: *Snores.*

I spend a lot of time during the first lockdown expressing relief that I am sober. 'Thank GOD I don't drink anymore,' I say again and again to Harry, and I mean it, I really do. If I was still drinking when the pandemic hit – assuming I had managed to stay alive until the pandemic hit, that is – I almost certainly would have killed myself with booze and drugs within the first few weeks of the lockdown. The sun. The weirdness. The sense that the world was perhaps ending and all normal rules were out, so fuck it, why not sit in the garden getting pissed? I would have drunk myself into a stupor by day two.

Some days, I imagine particularly detailed scenarios that might have happened were I still drinking and using drugs. Being caught sneaking out to meet a dealer, and getting thrown in prison. My child being taken away from me because I was incapable of looking after her. Before I found myself in rehab, the only things keeping me from complete and utter alcoholic oblivion were the structures of everyday life: the need to take my child to nursery or be in an office by a certain time. I didn't always manage to achieve these things – quite often, Harry would have to do nursery drop-off, while I lay in bed stewing in my own sweat and self-loathing, trying to cook up a new and original excuse for why I was going to be late for work – but the knowledge of them kept me vaguely on track. Without these structures, I dread to think what would have happened to me. And yet now, in these early days of the pandemic, I *do* think about what would have happened. I think about it all the time. Not in a grim, macabre way, but in a way that makes me feel profoundly relieved that I managed to get sobriety pre-Covid.

I am just over two and a half years sober when the pandemic starts. Two and a half years without a drink sounds like a long time, doesn't it? But I am discovering that, in emotional terms, it is like being a two-and-a-half-year-old child. When you have been numbing your feelings for decades, the rediscovery of them in sobriety can sometimes make life feel like one long toddler tantrum. Perhaps this explains the strangeness of my behaviour, the weird inability I have to acknowledge that I seem to have switched out one problem for another.

So I go to twelve-step meetings online, and I listen and I nod along as we all express our gratitude for having a programme, for not needing to drink. But even though I don't need to drink, that doesn't mean I don't *want* to drink. That I don't envy the people who can. I know it would be a disaster if I picked up a can of beer, but I can't help feeling a tiny bit of jealousy when I think about all the people sitting in their gardens, blocking out the madness of the world with rosé instead of raw chorizo. One night, when the rules have been slightly relaxed and people are allowed to meet in public spaces in small groups, I sit in the living room in the late spring–early summer heat with the windows open, trying not to think about the people drinking in the park down the road. Instead, I listen to a late-night meeting on Zoom, with attendees from as far afield as Sydney and New York, all of us alcoholics trying to stay sober during a pandemic. I lie on the sofa and I find myself chanting the words, 'I am sober, I am sober, I am sober,' over and over again, both an incantation of gratitude and a reminder to myself that however wrong I feel deep inside, at least I'm not drinking anymore.

I'm not sure how long I lie there, wittering away like the lunatic I have proven myself to be time and time again. But at some point, I am interrupted by the sound outside of a woman, drunkenly slurring insults into the air.

'You are always in the way!' She shrieks so loudly that I briefly look out the window to see what the commotion is about. Her hair is skew-whiff and her make-up is smeared, but from the neck down she appears completely normal: Birkenstock sandals, long swishy skirt, a T-shirt. Thirty seconds pass before I realise who she is talking to: a small, sobbing boy aged no more than seven or eight, who lags behind, begging her to wait for him.

'Mummy, please, I love you,' he chokes, as she staggers from one side of the pavement to the other, clearly returning home from the local common after too many hours of drinking, perhaps with other friends with children.

I am horrified. I think about going outside and intervening, but I am ashamed to say that feelings of hypocrisy stop me. What could I possibly say? What could I possibly do? And anyway, before I can do anything, they have disappeared from view, round a corner, on to another street, leaving me only with the knowledge that in another life and another world, that woman could have been me.

'I am sober, I am sober, I am *sober*,' I repeat to myself, a prayer for that woman and her son as much as it is for me. I sneak into the kitchen and find some more chorizo and beef jerky. I am so relieved that I am free of booze and drugs that I don't seem to realise I have fallen face-down into my first addiction: food.

Long before cocaine, long before ale and beer and Cava and bad men and Marlboro Golds, there were Herta frankfurters.

You know the ones: long, thin, beige, chemically processed, vacuum-packed into plastic, with that weird bit of water at the bottom.

What *was* that water?

It doesn't matter.

Yum.

Some children get told off for eating too many sweets and chocolate, but that wasn't an option for me.

The sweets were kept in a Winnie-the-Pooh tin on a shelf that was unreachable even by my mother – even if I had climbed on to a chair to get at them, it would have been far too obvious a crime, sweets being the go-to of most humans under the age of twelve. And let me tell you now: as a child growing up in the eighties, I had learned that eating sweet things was absolutely a crime, one punishable with any number of the horrible diets to which my mother and her friends subjected themselves: the cabbage soup diet; the cottage cheese diet; the grapefruit diet; and so on and so forth until you wasted away to some arbitrary size that seemed to change as often as the direction of the wind. These diets were supplemented by Jane Fonda workout videos – 'Go for the burn!' commanded Jane, from the tiny, flickering box TV in the corner of the living room that was the height of technology at the time.

So I always knew that I was never going to get away with scoffing sweet things in the quantities my anxious brain craved. Here, then, was the first sign that I had been born an addict: my cravings already thought they could outsmart the society around them. Sweets weren't going to cut it, but I needed *something* to fill the space in my stomach that I now see was actually the massive hole in my soul. And the thing that worked, for the early years of my life, was the salty deliciousness of Herta frankfurters.

How did it come to this? Let me explain. When I was growing up, we had a sixties-style fridge. I remember that it looked pretty cool, and that the coolness of the outside of the fridge was sadly not a reflection of the coolness of its inside. 'Style over substance' just about summed up my childhood home: everything looked lovely, but absolutely nothing worked.

So the beautiful fridge was always breaking, leaving our family with an almost constant need to consume large amounts of food so it wouldn't go to waste. My father said this happened because he was Jewish. Not the fridge breaking, you understand – it was not an antisemitic fridge – but the need to not let anything go to waste. 'Do you think our people suffered so that we could just throw this taramasalata in the bin?' he would exclaim, waving a bright pink tub in the air. 'Now eat!'

I don't know why it never occurred to my dad that it would be far less wasteful to throw away the old fridge and get a new one that didn't break every three days. I also don't know why, given his Jewish heritage, the broken fridge was often loaded with Herta frankfurters. Perhaps my mother, who is not Jewish, had convinced him they were made from some sort of pork substitute? Perhaps he is one of those annoying people who only invoke their faith when it enables them to make a point? Either way, these strange circumstances provided the perfect foil for my addiction to Herta frankfurters. Frankfurterism, if you will.

I didn't know that I was showing all the classic signs of addiction, because I was only six or seven and I had yet to be marched into a dark, dank community hall and forced to listen to a reformed drug addict talk about all the ways in which he was powerless over crack cocaine, and how it had made his life unmanageable. But there I was, not yet in double digits, and already displaying some pretty tell-tale symptoms of hopeless drug dependency – it just happened to be that the drug in question was an ultra-processed food available on supermarket shelves, rather than a substance procured in dark alleyways and smoked off tin foil.

Signs of addiction (feel free to replace the word 'frankfurters' with alcohol/cocaine/gambling/sex/shopping, etc., etc.)

Obsessive thoughts and actions, whereby acquiring and eating Herta frankfurters becomes the main priority in life, while almost all other obligations, including family and school, are sidelined.

Check! Sometimes, my fantasies about Herta frankfurters were such that at the weekend, while playing in my bedroom with my Sylvanian Families, I could almost hear the uncooked sausages calling to me from the fridge in the kitchen. 'Eat us, Bryony!'

49

cried the little Herta frankfurters, from underneath a packet of chicken breasts. 'Eat us!' And then I would be forced to sneak downstairs, checking the coast was clear, and peer into the fridge, where I would pretend I was looking for a carton of apple juice if anybody happened to catch me.

Disregard of harm caused, so that although the frank- furter use is causing physical and mental distress to the individual and/or their loved ones, the person struggling with addiction continues using frankfurters.

Check! Though I was only young, I wasn't stupid. I had a mother who would cling all day to a can of Diet Coke for sustenance. Thanks to her obsessive dieting (which was entirely normal back then), I knew that Herta frankfurters, in the volume I ate them, were not good for you. That they would possibly end up causing me to be the very worst thing it was possible for a woman to be: fat. Once, my mother had nibbled on one of my frankfurters during dinner, and then scolded herself for her naughtiness. 'Bad me, eating a bit of your frankfurter – eating any frankfurter at all!' Her tone was jokey and light, as if she was chastising a small child, that small child being herself. But I read from it the correct message: to overeat was to err. And if this was the case, I was erring all the time.

Despite this knowledge, I couldn't stop. I wouldn't stop. I didn't want to be the kind of girl who did unladylike things, such as eating huge quantities of frankfurters, and yet, try as I might, I couldn't stop myself from eating huge quantities of frankfurters. If they were there, I would have them, and nothing – nothing at all – could prevent me from making that happen.

*Loss of control, so that even in the face of
wanting to stop or reduce their frankfurter use,
the person cannot do so.*

Check! I mean, this one requires no further comment, really.

*Denial of addiction, so that when confronted,
the person battling addiction will deny or downplay
their frankfurter consumption. In order to avoid
having to explain themselves to others, the person
may consume frankfurters in secret.*

Check, check, check!

Once, my mother found two empty Herta frankfurters packets
hidden under my bed. I don't know how long the slimy containers
had remained there, but they had obviously started to smell,
causing my mother to carry out a huge search while I was away
at a sleepover. I remember getting home, tired from staying up
until 11pm eating sweets (sweets were not frankfurters, sadly),
and my mother producing the packets from an old Tesco bag in
the fridge, as if conjuring a rabbit out of a hat.

'What on earth are *these* doing in your bedroom?' she questioned, as if she had found actual drugs in the room of her
eight-year-old daughter. I felt adrenaline course through me. How
was I going to get out of this one? At that moment, our labrador,
Polo, leapt at my mother and the empty frankfurter packets. The
universe had provided me with a helpful excuse in canine form.

'I don't know, maybe blame him!' I started to cry, already
able to manipulate the situation like a master addict. 'Why
would I be hiding empty frankfurter packets in my bedroom?
That's gross!'

Then my mother came and held me in her arms, the slimy packets now being licked completely clean by Polo, while she dabbed away at my tears. 'I wasn't telling you off, darling,' she said. 'I just wanted to understand why there was a health and safety risk developing in your bedroom, that's all. Bad Polo, bad boy!' I snuggled into her, and for the first time in my life, I felt the blessed addict's relief of getting away with something.

What was I trying to change? What fears already had me in such a vice-like grip that I needed to eat cold, heavily processed meat in an attempt to try and vanquish them? I could list the anxieties that plagued my childhood in the same way that other kids could list games they liked to play: the house could burn down and it would be all my fault for not raising the alarm in time; there could be a downpour of acid rain that would burn off all of our skin, and it would be all my fault for not alerting my family to the dangers of using products made from burning fossil fuels; in the unlikely event that the acid rain didn't burn off all of our skin, it could still come down in such large amounts that it would cause a flood that would drown us, and it would be all my fault for not alerting my family to the dangers of deforestation in the Amazon; the hole in the ozone layer could get so big that we would all boil to death, and it would be all my fault because I hadn't done enough to stop people from using CFCs.

I think that just about covers it.

'A worrier': that was how my mum described me. 'You worry when you've got nothing to worry about,' she observed, not entirely unfairly. But 'worrier' was one of those words that was doing quite a lot of heavy lifting in the eighties and nineties – like 'troubled' and 'difficult', it was a word people used to describe a human who didn't fit into the narrow respectability mould that had been made at some Victorian factory in the late nineteenth century. I don't blame my parents at all for this – they were simply using a vocabulary that had probably been used on them by their parents, who in turn had had it used on them by theirs – but I do now know that I was more than just a worrier. I was really unwell. I was in an almost permanent state of terror. I have precious few carefree, happy memories of childhood, though this was not for a lack of trying on my parents' behalf. They loved me, and they wanted the best for me; they just did not live in a society that knew how to handle anything other than 'normal' and 'good'.

Nothing about my upbringing could explain my mental illness. There was nothing that was done to me, nothing I had experienced, that might have caused me to be so troubled, and such a worrier. My parents appeared happy; they loved us; we had a comfortable life in a comfortable house; I went to a private school, where I was neither bullied nor a bully; there was a Volvo Estate; there were frequent wholesome holidays to the beach in Cornwall. And yet, despite all this apparent privilege, I knew there was something not quite right with me. I felt odd. I felt other. I felt, somehow, *mad*. I couldn't explain it or articulate it as a seven- to eight-year-old. I couldn't really articulate it as a twenty-seven-year-old, or even as a thirty-seven-year-old; perhaps I will still be trying to articulate it as a forty-seven-year-old. But it was already there in the atmosphere around me: the knowledge that I was not as I was supposed to be, and that because of this, something terrible was about to happen.

I know from talking to other people who have experienced mental illness that this feeling of being other is not actually that unusual at all. That it is, in fact, the most normal thing in the world to feel weird. But back then, I had no knowledge of the term 'mental health', much less what it entailed – and even if I had, I doubt that knowledge alone would have been enough to stop the powerful voice of Jareth, who likes to sit in my head and tell me that I don't have mental health issues at all, I'm just evil. But this, I have learned, is how mental illness thrives: by isolating you. By making you feel like a freak. By telling you that nobody else in the world is thinking what you're thinking. I had yet to discover that, actually, quite a lot of people were thinking what I was thinking; that there were hundreds if not thousands of kids my age eating away their feelings of otherness. I just thought I was bad. Faulty. Wrong. My very existence had created some sort of rip in the space–time continuum that would let in disaster and catastrophe for me and every single person I loved.

There were many ways, over the years, in which I tried to change my feeling of otherness, of being wrong. I tried to change it with the obsessive chanting and rumination of OCD that I believed would prove I wasn't bad. I tried to change it with the drink and drugs that would silence the voice of Jareth in my head. And I tried to change it with bulimia.

I was nineteen years old the first time I threw up a meal on purpose. At the time, I did not feel that I had developed an eating disorder, more that I had discovered a delicious secret. Here was the answer to my shameful love of food: I would simply sneak off after eating it, and force it all out of my system. With bulimia, I could enjoy all the narcotic, dream-like effects of a binge without feeling like a fat cow. And being a 'fat cow' was, after all, the very worst thing a young woman could be in the nineties and noughties – worse even than being judgemental, hateful and small-minded. Having a small mind when it came to weight did not matter. What mattered was a small waist.

Though I was not even close to being fat, it didn't matter. Fat was more a state of mind than a number on a scale.

'I'm so fat,' a friend would say, pinching at a bony hip.

'I'm just disgusting at the moment,' my mother's size-eight best mate would announce while round for a coffee ('No milk, thanks, I'm on a diet!').

The other day, I heard a perfectly slim TV presenter talking about her 'lifetime of weight issues' that she had 'finally' managed to get under control thanks to a juicing retreat she visited twice a year. I looked at this brilliant, successful woman, who has always, always seemed on the slight side to me, and I realised that her 'weight issues' weren't actually weight issues at all – they were issues implanted in each of us by the patriarchy to keep us, quite literally, small. To stop us from taking up space. If we are too busy being subjugated by fears of getting too big physically, then we will not have the energy to step into the hugeness of our female power mentally. But back then, I just saw thinness as a goal. As an achievement. As a way to make people like me more. If I looked good on the outside, then surely I would not feel so bad on the inside.

Eating disorders are not really about weight, as we all know – they are about control. But in a world obsessed with weight and body image, they are as good a way as any to try and get that control. And I had no control whatsoever, quite clearly. I was, in the terminology of tabloid culture at the time, completely out of control. Consider the way that female celebrities of the time were shamed on the covers of magazines for doing perfectly normal things like *existing*. To go out in the evening and be photographed leaving a club with your make-up slightly smudged and your hair not brushed was to be in the grips of a breakdown. To go on holiday and have a single fold of skin visible above your bikini bottoms was tantamount to checking out of polite society and giving up on life entirely. To appear messy, to not fit into our culture's incredibly narrow definition of female acceptability, was to be an abject failure. I knew this in the same way that I knew how to breathe. It was written into the very fabric of my DNA.

Messy, wild, feral: I was all of the very worst ways to be a woman. I knew this because I had heard people refer to their 'over-eating' – imbibing two squares of chocolate – and that just looked like 'eating' to me. If eating a bag of crisps was 'pigging out', then I was an entire team of wild boars, rampaging through the wilderness and snuffling up whatever they could get their snouts on. As I got older, my pudgy hands tore through frankfurters, pork pies and scotch eggs like tissue paper. I would eat yards and yards of pizza in one sitting, my attempts to numb out giving rise only to a terrible feeling of nausea. And if I felt sick, I reasoned, then I might as well *be* sick. It made sense. It made everything neater. It gave balance to something terribly skew-whiff. If I forced my index finger down my throat and purged after a binge, then I would be able to right all the wrongs in my world.

So my addiction to strange food was joined by an addiction to vomiting up that strange food. And as with all addictions, I had rules. When it came to my alcoholism, I would refuse to drink wine because it caused me to black out too quickly (clearly, wine was the problem, rather than the quantity and the speed at which I drank it). With bulimia, I had to eat my food in stages – vegetable, protein then carbohydrate – so that when I threw it up, I would know when I had got to the end. I could not wait for longer than ten minutes to purge – ten minutes being some arbitrary cut-off I had created in my mind, after which point all the calories would be absorbed into my body and I would prove myself to be the awful, fat cow I was.

But the problem with living like this is that after a while – a while being many, many years – it starts to take its toll on your body. Your teeth begin to fall out. Your throat begins to feel like sandpaper. Your skin gets sallow. But mostly, your soul begins to call out to you, and as it calls out to you, it asks you to stop. It says: 'For the sake of the mother you will become and the daughter you will have and the woman you deserve to be, please stop doing this to yourself. Please stop trying to disappear. Please stay, and stay exactly as you are. Please stop judging everything through a shattered and myopic lens that wants you to be something you're not. Please, just stop.'

So I did. When people ask me why I stopped being bulimic, and why I stopped hiding my body away, I tell them the truth: I stopped because I wanted to start living. I got angry that this was how I was expected to live my life, in a perpetual state of self-loathing. I got angry that the default setting for women and young girls was to put themselves down; that the biggest insult you could give a woman was that she was full of herself. And I decided, in my anger, to be full of myself. To be full of my power and my glory and my brilliance, and to stop behaving in ways that diminished me.

I stopped bingeing and purging. I put on weight. I filled out. I gave up trying to shrink myself, and fleshed out to the size-eighteen woman I firmly believe had been struggling to get out of my size-ten body all along. I treated my body like the complex set of systems it had always been, rather than a set of sewage pipes blocked by cooking fat, make-up wipes and tampons.

I realised that I was not a fat cow. I was a unique, worthy human being who had every right to be here, exactly as I wanted to be – small, big, hairy, waxed, and everything in between. I discovered that the odds of any of us existing were one in 102,685,000. That there was literally more chance of dinosaurs roaming the earth again.

Evidence that you are a miracle

- On the day you were conceived, a single sperm beat millions of other sperms in the equivalent of a sperm Ironman challenge, in order to fertilise an egg that would only have been there for a couple of calendar days each month.
- That egg was surrounded by white blood cells that behaved like nightclub bouncers, stopping any riff-raff getting in.
- If your biological father had said something annoying to your biological mother, or the door bell had gone, a different sperm might have made it to the egg and created a different version of you!
- Instead, it created the zygote that would become you. And as we know, sadly, not every zygote goes the distance.
- The day you are born is considered by the majority of doctors to be one of the most dangerous of your life. And you survived it.
- You have gone on to survive every day since. And if you are anything like me (which I imagine you might be, because you bought this book), that's kind of a miracle in itself. You haven't been killed by alcoholism or addiction or an eating disorder or depression. You are an absolute fucking stone-cold miracle. The universe really, really wants you here, and it wants you here exactly as you are. Not looking like a fitness influencer or a Kardashian or a Hadid, but as yourself.

I decided then to embrace my body instead of rejecting it. To remind everyone that they are a glorious gift to the planet that absolutely deserves to be here.

I ran a marathon in my pants, and then got 700 women to run ten kilometres through the streets of London in theirs. I started posting unfiltered pictures of myself on Instagram, ones that showed off my cellulite rather than hiding it. I became an accidental ambassador for body positivity, though really the term I prefer is body acceptance. I wasn't the kind of person telling others to stand in the mirror saying they love themselves – I just wanted them to stop standing there listing all the ways they hated themselves.

I am asked all the time how I got my confidence, how I can freely be so happy in my body after being so very unhappy in it for so long. I wish I could distil my answer into a neat paragraph, one you could cut out and keep in your wallet for every time you feel low and need a little pep talk. But life doesn't work like that. There is no simple answer to what happened, although I can try and sum it up as simply as possible: I had a child; I saw the magic of my body; I started eating normally; I stopped drinking and taking drugs; I discovered that exercise was not about the losses, but the gains, and that if I did it for how it made me feel rather than how it made me look, I became a whole lot more self-accepting.

But mostly, I 'got my confidence' because I got fed up. It wasn't so much that I suddenly felt great all the time, more that I became tired of feeling *bad* all the time. I didn't develop confidence, just a desire not to spend another moment of my precious life hating on myself.

4

Chorizo blackout

Snapshot from my iPhone's Notes App, November 2020

< Notes   ⬆ ⋯

Ice cream (by Edie)

I love ice cream

So cold so soft

It's so yummy in my tummy

I cover you in sprinkles

I sing a nice song

It gives me a brain frees

I give you a hug then I eat you up

I love 💕 ice 🎁 cream

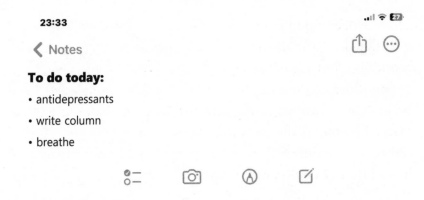

To do today:

• antidepressants

• write column

• breathe

Almost exactly a year after our trip to Thailand, I wake up with a familiar and shocking feeling, one I have not felt now for 1,191 days, or 28,584 hours, or 1,715,040 minutes.

I have a hangover.

It's just that this time, it's a food hangover.

The physical sensations are all the same. My head is fuzzy, my throat is drier than the Gobi desert, and my body feels leaden. The emotions, too, are startlingly similar. There is shame, there is regret, there is the sense that I can never, ever feel this way again. And, like a hangover caused by alcohol, there is a lag between me coming round and me piecing together the events that have led to this overwhelming sense of dread. I am familiar with the concept of blacking out because of drink, but until now, I hadn't realised you could also do it with *food*.

I prop myself up in bed and become aware that I am soaked through with sweat. My nightie is sodden. There is a horribly sweet, decaying smell in the air, and I realise it is coming from me. I turn to my right and see that instead of my husband lying in bed next to me, there are two empty packets of pork scratchings, one bright green tube of sour cream and onion Pringles and eight packets of Hula Hoops. Not quite the strangest situation

I have woken up in after a binge – it's probably best I don't get
into the time a man tried to use a tub of Lurpak on me as a
lubricant – but it's definitely up there.

I shudder at the crumbs on the sheets, the ones that must
be mingling with my sweat, and the vague memory of lying to
Harry hits me in the stomach. It has been a long time since I
fibbed to my husband in order to fuel an addiction. I used to
lie to him so I could drink more – 'I'm just going to stay downstairs and clean up!' I would trill as he went to bed, painting
a picture of me as some sort of Mary Poppins figure, when in
fact I was more like Alan in *The Hangover*, 'secretly' hoovering
up lines of cocaine and bottles of beer as if my beloved was a
non-sentient being who wouldn't notice his wife not coming
to bed until 6am.

But last night, I lied to him so I could eat more.

'I think I've got a cold coming on,' I remember telling him at
midnight, making the 'helpful' suggestion that he should go and
sleep in the spare room so as not to 'catch' whatever it is I have
(a binge eating disorder, as it will turn out). He got up, shuffled
off, and I felt the jolt of elation that was knowing I could eat
whatever I wanted without the shame of being caught.

That elation was short-lived. It always is. You're always chasing
another hit, one that's surely just around the corner, found in the
substance or process that you happen to be addicted to: alcohol,
drugs, sex, shopping, gambling, food.

I remember creeping downstairs and opening the fridge, only
to be met with the crushing disappointment that was no chorizo.
I was furious with myself, filled with the type of anger I usually
reserve for the government, or those dicks on GB News. How
could it have been that just that morning, I had *really and truly*
believed that I wasn't going to binge again? In that state of

complete and utter delusion, I had failed to go to Sainsbury's and restock. And now, I was standing there in the cold, harsh light of the fridge, realising what an absolute asshat I'd been.

The lack of chorizo might have deterred other, less addicted people from their midnight fridge raid. It might have resulted in nothing more than a shrug of the shoulders and a return to bed. But I was on a mission. I had begun the process of a binge, and – as all good addicts know – once a binge has been started, the only way it can be stopped is by reaching complete and utter oblivion. Without my primary addiction, what was I to numb myself with? I scanned the fridge for other readily edible food. All good night-bingers know that you can't start preparing and cooking food when you should be soundly asleep in your bed, because with the clatter of pots and pans, everyone – yourself included – would know there was a problem. I stared forlornly into the practically empty chasm of our American-style fridge freezer, the type I used to see in sitcoms as a child, and then later fantasise about, because in them I imagined such a dizzying array of snackable, beige food, I would never be in any danger of being found out. The reality was a little different that dark, tedious night at some point during lockdown number two. The fridge contained: a jar of mustard; half a pint of milk; a carton of apple juice; a piece of plastic cheese that had been there since a barbecue we'd held in the summer of 2019, back when we were innocent and naive and actually able to socialise; some uncooked salmon (for some reason, I have always drawn a line at raw fish, as if I am some sort of civilised human being and not a savage who rips through raw spiced sausage with her bare teeth); a cucumber; some spinach; a courgette; two ageing carrots. The vegetables stared back at me, the equivalent of an alcoholic being offered a glass of water instead of a shot of vodka. I grabbed the plastic cheese in an attempt to sate the rage I was feeling at the fridge's scant offerings, and then I moved to the cupboard.

The sight of the Pringles genuinely left me feeling as high as any line of cocaine ever could. I would have let out a whoop, were it not for the fact that I was a forty-year-old woman lost in the depths of a tragic food spiral while her daughter and husband slumbered quietly upstairs, no doubt dreaming the dreams of innocents whose only desire was to be able to socialise indoors, with someone they didn't already live with. I grabbed the Pringles, in the same fevered way I used to grab a pint at the bar. Then I saw the Hula Hoops, and the pork scratchings, and like some demented cross between a child in a sweet shop and a darts player in a pub, I shoved the items up my nightie and tiptoed my way back upstairs.

The rest of the night was a blur, an endless cycle of eating and numbing and shame, followed by more eating and numbing and shame. When I ran out of the food from the cupboard, I started thinking about the food in the bin. The leftovers scraped from our plates just a few hours earlier. The soggy, half-eaten fish finger my seven-year-old couldn't finish, the fat trimmed from the steak that my husband had refused to eat. I crept back downstairs, placed my foot on the pedal of the bin, and reached inside.

And it was at this point, I think, that I entered blackout.

Cross-addiction for dummies

Cross-addiction, which is also known as 'addiction transfer', is when you swap one addiction for another. It is different from dual addiction, which is when someone has more than one addiction at the same time (for example, alcohol and cocaine).

Cross-addiction is very common in people in early sobriety from alcohol and drugs. When I was in rehab, cross-addiction to cigarettes was rife – in fact, an addiction to nicotine was seen as the lesser of two evils, and it was suggested by a counsellor to 'deal with whatever is going to kill you first'. For some people, that was alcohol and drugs; for others, it was food. Everyone is different.

Common cross addictions include sex (this is why new relationships are discouraged in early sobriety), food, gambling, gaming and shopping.

There are many dozens of twelve-step fellowships, modelled on the original programme of Alcoholics Anonymous, that help people to recover from addictive processes. These include Debtors Anonymous, Overeaters Anonymous, Gamblers Anonymous, Sex and Love Addicts Anonymous, and Codependents Anonymous.

If at night, I am a deranged bin-raider, by day, I am a respectable mental health campaigner, the founder of a national peer-support group called Mental Health Mates, and an award-winning columnist at a broadsheet newspaper. People come to me for advice. They look to me for wise counsel. I have never been as sought after as I am during this pandemic; my ability to deal with the bin fire of addiction, OCD and depression seems to have turned me into some sage that people come to in the hope that I might be able to solve whatever ails them. My inbox and my social media DMs boil over with messages from people telling me about their problems, about their inability to stop drinking, or their terrible OCD that has left them wrapped in the horror of their own heads for weeks. These messages mean a lot to me. But they also, inadvertently, remind me of what a fraud I am. A weak, gluttonous fraud who is incapable of practising what she preaches.

At some point during the first lockdown, my publisher suggests that I write a practical guide to mental health, as it might help people struggling with theirs at this difficult time. I agree, and set about writing all the things about mental wellness that I could only have learned from experiencing mental illness. But as I approach the end of the book, I don't feel a sense of achievement. I just see the huge disconnect between the woman who spends her days interviewing experts on how to spot psychosis, and the one who spends her nights out of her mind eating chorizo.

I tell myself that it is just the stress of writing a book. That's all this is. And it's not as if I am throwing up any of the food I am eating, so I can't be that bad, can I? In fact, if you look at it that way, I am basically winning at life. I am bingeing, but not purging! I am a shining beacon of recovery!

These delusions fuel me for a few hours of each day, enabling me to get my work done. But then at 4pm, I am back to thinking about dinner. And snacks. And chorizo. A battle takes place in my head: a battle between a part of me that thinks I'm a snivelling, self-indulgent so-and-so for making an issue out of chorizo when there's a deadly pandemic raging outside, and the one who just wants that other part of me to shut the fuck up, and only knows how to do this by numbing themselves with food. To complicate matters further, my husband seems to have turned into Sylvester Stallone. He has gone on a health and fitness drive, I think as a way of coping with being stuck inside with me all day. If he's not working, he is in the living room, lifting weights and grunting, or concocting a meal that involves lean protein and vegetables. His favourite seems to be turkey balls with cauliflower 'mash'.

'How about I make it tonight for both of us?' he asks one day, and the idea fills me with such rage that I actually tell him to fuck off.

'Why would I want that?! How can you suggest I go on a diet? If I wasn't married to you, I'd cancel you!'

He doesn't mention it again.

I wonder: when will my way of coping involve plentiful exercise and healthy food, as opposed to raw sausages and McCoy's cheddar and onion crisps? The shame doubles – as, I'm sure, has my waistline. But to worry about this seems like a terrible deception, a rejection of the values I espouse so passionately in my writing and on social media. Surely, by now, I, of all people, should have managed to free myself from the shackles of diet culture? And so the shame doubles again: I feel shame for feeling shame.

One day, while Harry is out on a casual twenty-one-kilometre run, an Amazon driver arrives bearing a box for my husband. Without thinking, I open it. Inside, I find a set of brand new, gleaming digital scales, the type that measure visceral fat and hydration levels, and only just stop short of looking into your soul. I have not stood on a scale for years now, preferring not to judge my value by a measure of weight. It has taken me years to view myself as a human, rather than a dress size. But something has shifted inside me without me realising it. I can't pinpoint exactly when it happened, but at some stage between the start of the first lockdown and now, the second one, I seem to have abandoned all my principles, the ones that kept me safe from disordered eating.

I stand on the scales.

I feel a stab of revulsion familiar to me from my days of bulimia.

I run to the corner shop, where I begin the process of losing myself in several large grab bags of cheese and onion crisps.

On the plus side: there is still no sign of Jareth.

I have decided that I want the central part of my new book to be a guide to how to get emergency help when you are in a mental health crisis. I have a theory that the more ingrained this knowledge is in the population, the more the government will have to provide proper funding to services. We all know what to do if we break a leg, or if our child has a fever for more than a couple of days – go to A&E. But what if we are feeling suicidal? What if we are incapable of leaving the house because of obsessions and compulsions and generalised anxiety? How do we find help then? There have been more than a couple of occasions in my life when I have found myself in crisis, unsure of what to do, and if *I'm* unsure of what to do, despite my years of work in this area, what hope does anyone else have?

I have another theory, too. Although it is important to highlight and raise awareness around the lack of mental health provision out there, I think that endlessly hearing about said lack probably has an unintended consequence, in that it puts people off looking for help. In focusing on what *isn't* available, we can sometimes miss what *is*. And despite the lack of funding, there are some excellent examples of mental healthcare in the UK. I decide that I want my new book to contain a comprehensive guide to these examples, with advice on how best to navigate a system that can be deeply confusing to the uninitiated.

To do this, I interview paramedics and people who work in

71

Child and Adolescent Mental Health Services. I interview GPs and psychotherapists and volunteers for the Samaritans. I also interview Naomi, an expert on eating disorders.

'I don't know much about eating disorders,' I say, in my opening to Naomi, and I immediately realise that this is a lie, one I am too ashamed to correct. Then I start asking her about signs and symptoms and treatment plans, and how to help your child if they are suffering from anorexia or bulimia.

'I should also say that while it's important to focus on anorexia and bulimia, we shouldn't forget that the most common eating disorder in the UK and US is actually binge eating disorder.' Naomi pauses here, and I feel something strange pass through my whole body, something like clarity.

'Is that when you binge food but you don't purge it?' I ask.

'Yes. People often think that if they aren't purging or restricting their food, then they can't have an eating disorder. But that's not the case. Binge eating disorder involves consuming very large amounts of food without feeling as if you have any control. You can't stop. We think it affects about three times the number of people diagnosed with anorexia nervosa and bulimia nervosa combined, and yet we don't really hear about it enough. If you could mention it in the book, you'd be really helping us out.'

'I think I can do that,' I say, feeling tears fall down my cheeks.

'That would be great,' says Naomi. 'You're a star.'

You wouldn't say that if you knew me, I think. *You wouldn't say that at all.*

5

I think I might be pregnant with an alien

Snapshot from my iPhone's Notes App, December 2020

< Notes

Gratitude list

- having husband who can do fiendishly complicated maths with Edie
- not having had Covid
- new series of *Mandalorian*
- Pedro Pascal
- my skin is really good at the moment???

I think five things is enough, don't you?

I had always thought of the word 'binge' as denoting a very British kind of guilty pleasure. A bit naughty, but a bit fun, too. Binge drinking. Binge watching. Binge eating. The kind of thing we know we 'shouldn't' do, but we allow ourselves to do because life's too short – and why would the universe create vodka, Netflix and crisps if it didn't want us to consume them in large quantities? We live in a binge culture, a culture of *more*, and yet, after finishing my interview with Naomi, I am left with the distinct feeling that the word 'binge' might just have developed a more sinister meaning to me. One that has more in common with addiction.

In the coming weeks and months, I will learn that for me, as an alcoholic in recovery, there is an ever-so-thin line between bingeing on something for fun, and being addicted to it out of necessity. And with food, I have well and truly crossed that line.

Actually, I haven't just crossed it. I have trekked such a distance from it that I am now essentially lost in the world of food addiction, my camp set up in its wildest, most dangerous mountains: just me, my tent and a lifetime's supply of chorizo and cheese and onion crisps. Binge eating disorder this may be, but make no mistake – it is also food addiction, by another name.

The relief of knowing that I have a classifiable problem is quickly replaced by the knowledge that I now have to do something about this classifiable problem. And I am, quite frankly, fed up with having to do something about classifiable problems. OCD, depression, bulimia, alcoholism and now this? As a child, I had somewhat naively believed that 'happy' was an ending, a destination, a place you made a mighty effort to get to and then, having made that effort, you got to stay there for the rest of your life. Now I am seeing that it is more of a moveable feast, the emotional equivalent of winning an Olympic gold medal and immediately having to start training for the European Championships.

'I can't believe there's something *else* wrong with me,' I tell Peter, in our next session. 'I am forty years old and still discovering new things about myself that are faulty.'

I laugh, as if performing some sort of comedy sketch.

'From what you've said, Bryony, binge eating isn't new to you.' He looks so earnest, so unwilling to join me in my performance. 'It sounds as if food was actually the first thing you ever got addicted to.'

A comfortable silence cloaks the room as I let that sink in for a bit. Progress, then: just a couple of years ago, I would have rushed to fill that silence, the idea of sitting in it being akin to sitting on a bed of nails or hot coals.

A memory comes to me unbidden, of going to Chessington World of Adventures for my twelfth birthday. It should have been a joyous moment, a fun moment, a moment of excitement and candy floss and Professor Burp's Bubbleworks. But I was miserable that day. I was miserable, because I had just turned twelve and I was sure I was pregnant. No matter that I was a virgin, and that my periods hadn't even started, I was convinced that there was something inside me, something evil that would ruin my life, something I had to get out of me by any means possible.

Anyway, it didn't matter that I was a virgin, because I was actually pregnant with a parasitic extra-terrestrial that had been placed in my body as I slept. Stop laughing at the back. I had been sure of this for a couple of months, ever since accidentally seeing a trailer for the film *Alien 3*, in which Sigourney Weaver reprised her role as Lieutenant Ripley, the kick-ass protagonist who travels through hyperspace to battle a terrifying species of monster with acid for blood and the ability to impregnate you by jumping on to your face and then bursting out of your chest. I was not, of course, old enough to see this film, but I had somehow caught a clip during an episode of *Wogan*, the early evening chat show that was a bit like *The One Show*, only with Terry Wogan instead of Ronan Keating (oh, how things were better in my day, et cetera, et cetera). The trailer was run just before an interview with Sigourney Weaver. Having accidentally seen the trailer – which featured a giant alien bursting through a canteen ceiling and devouring a man innocently eating his dinner – I became convinced that there were aliens living in the attic, the attic that I slept directly underneath, and that they were impregnating me in the night, without me knowing.

My body, then, was a ticking time bomb, but there was no way I could explain this to my parents or friends, who would have thought I was . . . mad. So I kept the secret tight inside my chest, with my baby alien, who was surely about to burst out and kill me at any moment. The only way to stop it was to kill it, but how? I had no idea what an abortion was, and that was probably just as well, because had I turned up to the doctor and asked them to terminate the alien inside me, I almost certainly would have been bundled off and locked away for the rest of my life, that being the predominant way to deal with anyone who showed even vague signs of mental disturbance in the nineties. This being quite an *extreme* sign of mental disturbance.

I had an idea, though. It involved going to a theme park, specifically Chessington World of Adventures, where I knew that – along with people under 1.1 metres, those suffering from heart conditions and anyone with a bad back – pregnant women were not allowed to go on the Vampire roller coaster, presumably because its high-speed twists and turns were dangerous for unborn babies. And aliens. This, then, was the perfect way to kill the creature inside me. I would ride the Vampire all day, and though aliens could survive hyperspace and Hollywood, this alien wouldn't stand a chance at a theme park just off the Leatherhead Road.

But how to organise a trip to Chessington World of Adventures, a special treat reserved only for birthdays? If the alien could just stay put until I turned twelve, I might be in with a chance of carrying out my plan, and then I would be saved (as would everyone around me, who would surely be killed by the alien as soon as it burst out of my chest at the kitchen table).

Miraculously, the alien stayed put, and did not burst out of my chest. And so it was that I remember my twelfth birthday not because of the fun that was had, but because I spent five hours of it repeatedly queuing to go on the Vampire roller coaster so I could see off the monster that lived inside me. While my friends begged to go on something else – the Magic Carpet, perhaps, or the log flume – I knew that only the endless corkscrews of the Vampire would finish off the alien foetus growing within me. At the end of the day, I got home and felt truly safe for the first time since I had seen the trailer for *Alien 3*. I was no longer pregnant with an alien, and all was well again.

Or at least, all was well until a couple of months later, when I would experience what I believe was my 'first' episode of OCD – the one that involved me becoming convinced that I had AIDS.

I haven't thought about my alien baby at all since it happened. Until now, it has never even occurred to me as being particularly weird – I'd just chalked it up to being one of those strange, almost-adolescent things that happened as you started to go through puberty and learn about the birds and the bees. But as Peter talks about food being my primary addiction, as he references the Herta frankfurters and the fact that I have been trying to numb my feelings from a very early age, it is as if my brain is waking up from a deep, deep slumber, finally acknowledging how long my body has felt ... well, *alien* to me. This wasn't something that started in my late teens or early twenties with the bulimia. It had been there all along, with the binge eating and the OCD and the strange beliefs I'd had that there might be aliens inside me.

Other signs from childhood that maybe everything was really not fine

- I preferred Benylin to Calpol, because it tasted stronger.
- I was given an inhaler even though I didn't have asthma, because I kept finding I couldn't breathe.
- I once locked my sister in a cupboard until she learned all the names of New Kids On The Block off by heart, and their birthdays.

I tell Peter the story about the pregnancy I believed with all my heart to be true, and how it has only just occurred to me that, actually, I was experiencing delusional thinking. I was, essentially, psychotic. He nods along, and I start to cry. How could I have forgotten this? How could I have failed to realise it before? And what has caused it to come up now?

'I've had an epiphany!' I exclaim, at the end of my rant, knowing that therapists love a bit of an epiphany – it is literally the whole reason they sit and listen to people wang on about their problems for many hours, the equivalent of seeing a teacher witness a previously failing pupil suddenly understanding quadratic equations. 'The monster inside me I was afraid of wasn't some terrifying Hollywood blockbuster alien.' I pause for dramatic effect, so we can both really savour this moment. 'It was *me*. My inherent badness. The inherent badness that I have been trying to solve through my OCD all these years, but which has only ever made me feel worse.'

I close my eyes and shake my head in a sort of astounded awe at my ability to psychoanalyse myself. When I open them, I see Peter beaming back at me, and I feel like his star pupil.

'Lots of people say that getting sober is like being handed the keys to the kingdom,' he explains. 'So often, we think that stopping drinking or getting clean is going to be the end of our lives. But actually, it's the start of them. Putting down alcohol is the first step, but it doesn't mean you're cured. The thing that made you pick up all that alcohol is still there, and that's you. Without the booze to numb it, you suddenly have to deal with yourself. With all the issues that were there all along, the ones you couldn't get to because you were too busy fighting to put out all the fires you had lit with your alcohol and cocaine use. It's not a surprise, really, that you've fallen head first into food, especially during one of the biggest collective traumas anyone has experienced in their lifetime. The only surprise to me is that it didn't happen sooner in your sobriety. You're not the first alcoholic to go into recovery and spend the first few years cross-addicting with other substances, and you won't be the last. For some, it's cigarettes. For others, it's sex. For you, it's food.'

Suddenly, I don't feel quite as clever.

'Actually, Peter, it's all three for me. I still smoke like a trooper, and I shan't go into all the masturbation that took place in the first year of my sobriety. So yes, I've cross-addicted to three

81

different things. I'm three and a bit years sober, and yet I'm behaving like a blind drunk.'

'You're here, acknowledging your problems. That seems like pretty grown-up behaviour to me. That seems like progress, even.'

'Why do you always do that?'

He tilts his head and raises his eyebrows quizzically. 'Do what, exactly, Bryony?'

'You know what,' I sigh. 'That *patronising* thing.' I cross my arms and look away from him out the window, like a sulky teenager who has gone from pleased-with-themselves to pissed-off-with-the-world at the flick of a switch.

'I'm sorry if that's your interpretation of what I am saying. That certainly wasn't my intention at all.' He is speaking calmly, and I feel like punching him for it.

Instead, I stay quiet and decide to play him at his own stupid therapist's game: the one where they say nothing, thus forcing the other person to do all the talking and revealing of their deepest, darkest secrets.

'If you don't mind me saying, you seem angry with me, Bryony.'

'URGHHH! There you go again! Being all reasonable! While I sit here collecting mental health problems as if they were Tesco Clubcard Points! OCD? That's fifty bonus points! Suicidal thoughts? Here's seventy-five points and ten quid off your next shop! Alcoholism? You have been entered into our special prize draw where everyone's a winner: binge eating, gambling, sex and love addiction! Which cross-addiction will you pick up and take home?'

'You're being very entertaining, as ever,' says Peter, not looking at all entertained. 'Do you feel that if you put on a show, you can avoid sitting and talking about the uncomfortable feelings that exist under these actions?'

'Peter, I am just trying to say that surely, *surely*, I should be a bit more *well* by this point of sobriety. By this point of life. God knows, I've done enough therapy. It just seems so bloody self-absorbed, given there's a bloody pandemic on and people are out there dying of *actual* illnesses. And here I am, still bleating about my stupid, petty little problems that never seem to go away.' I stop there and wince at the inbuilt ability I still have to gaslight myself, even as a so-called mental health campaigner who should know better than this. But it's hard, so, so hard.

'Bryony, you do know that all illness, mental or physical, isn't like mobile data, right?'

It's my turn to look confused.

'There's not a cap on how much you can have of it,' Peter says. 'You don't use it up, and then that's it for the rest of your life. You're a human, like any other. You have been incredibly unwell for a long time, and even with all the amazing work you've done – not just on yourself but in society, through your writing and your campaigning – you can't undo all those years of illness quickly. It takes time. Wellness is a journey like any other, with its own bumps, diversions and detours.'

'I can't believe you just did that,' I reply.

'Did what?'

'Used the words "wellness" and "journey" in one sentence. I think you just reached peak therapist.'

For the first time in our many months and years of working together, Peter actually rolls his eyes.

What your therapist says vs What they really mean

'You're quite enmeshed with your mother/father.'
They fuck you up, your mum and dad.
'Have you tried sitting with your feelings?'
Go right ahead and be a big old snotty mess, I've seen it all.
'Do you need a moment?'
You definitely need a moment.
'Have you heard of the concept of projecting?'
You're projecting.
'We're not here to talk about me.'
I see you trying to deflect this very difficult question I've just asked you
'Where did you go?'
Wow, you have totally disassociated.
'How is your inner child today?'
You're behaving like a three-year-old.

I reach out to Naomi again and ask for her help. Asking for help, as I have said many thousands of times, to many thousands of people, is the first and arguably most important step towards getting better. Why, then, do I feel like such a massive bell-end doing it? Is it the horrible sensation of shame I am feeling as I type out the message to Naomi, asking if she might be free for a quick chat to go over something I had missed during our first interview? I find myself closing my eyes as I tell her I think *I* have binge eating disorder, as if closing my eyes might suddenly give me an invisibility cloak and turn me into a character from the Marvel multiverse, thereby making me feel less embarrassed. Are there any Avengers whose special superpower is 'not feeling humiliated by one's own fallibility'? Have Chris

Hemsworth and Scarlett Johansson starred in that movie? If not, I think they should.

The point is: I *know* all this stuff about mental health. I know I shouldn't be embarrassed to admit I have a problem, that my brain is an organ like any other, and occasionally it might misfire. And yet, *knowing* this stuff doesn't seem to help. It doesn't stop it from happening to you – it just makes you feel even more stupid when it does. As I talk to Naomi, I feel a bit like someone who has a first from Oxbridge in Philosophy, Politics and Economics, but has just realised they don't actually know their times tables. After everything I've batted out the way, and all the body positivity work I've done, it seems kind of idiotic to find myself felled by binge eating disorder.

'Well nobody feels *clever* for developing an eating disorder,' says Naomi, not unreasonably. 'The feeling of shame you have is a symptom of BED in itself.'

As Naomi is a qualified eating disorders specialist, she explains that she can help me, in tandem with Peter. For some reason, I am embarrassed by this as well. It seems excessive to have a whole team to deal with my fucked-up brain, especially when so many others are struggling to access care. Who do I think I am? The Mariah fucking Carey of mental illness?

I mention this to Holly, one of my best friends. I met Holly in rehab. We have the same sobriety date. Though we have only known each other for three years, it feels like a lifetime, and perhaps that's because it is: getting sober *has* been the start of a whole new life for both of us. For Holly, it's also been the start of a whole new career. A year or so into her sobriety, she quit her job in advertising and began retraining as a psychotherapist. She is about to start a training placement at the very rehab where we met, and I am incredibly proud of her.

Holly and I check in every few days by phone, aware of the need for connection, especially in these strange times. 'Connection is the opposite of addiction!' she likes to remind me, as often as possible.

So I tell her about the binge eating, and the embarrassment, and the fact that it feels silly to have so many problems. When, oh when, will I be normal?

'Normal?' I can almost hear Holly spitting out her coffee on the other end of the phone. 'You of all people should know there's no such thing as normal.'

'No such thing as normal!' I beam. 'I like that. I might use that in a book one day, if you don't mind.'

'Go for it. Anyway, mate, if you think you've got problems, you should hear some of the stories I get told.' She laughs, her lightness immediately pricking my pompous feeling of self-importance. 'Obviously, for professional reasons, I can't share them with you, but believe me, a pinch of alcoholism, a dash of OCD and a soupçon of food issues is *nothing* compared to some of the chaos out there. Believe me when I say you're a shining beacon of sanity in a sea of people who can't even begin to acknowledge their problems. They don't want to look at them. They spend their entire lives doing everything they can to *not* look at them. They don't own any of their mess. They tell me again and again that they're not addicts, they're not alcoholics, they're not depressed, they're just fine. Fine. F-I-N-E.'

I stay quiet, but shudder at her mention of that word.

'If there's anything wrong with them,' she continues, 'it's everyone else's fault. It's their boyfriend's fault for cheating on them, or it's their dad's fault for being an arsehole, or it's their boss's fault for not promoting them. It's the fault of the barista in Pret A Manger for giving them a flat white with cow's milk when they clearly asked for oat milk. The whole world is against them, so of course they drink, of course they use drugs, of course they starve themselves or overeat or feel like absolute shit all the time, because who *wouldn't* in their circumstances?

'And you know, some of them have a point. A *lot* of them have a point. This world *is* fucking mental, and it's a wonder that more of us aren't in a perpetual state of breakdown. But there are some brave souls who decide they don't want to feel crap all the time. They don't want to have to numb themselves in order to survive. They know that survival is for people in war zones, for people who have been shipwrecked, for those really mad people who choose to trek up Everest. Survival is not a viable state when the biggest challenge of your day is whether or not to get lunch from Sainsbury's or M&S. So those brave souls – and they truly are brave souls, believe me – stand up and face whatever it is they are trying to survive. They stare it in the eyes, and they say, "No more! I don't want to live by surviving, I want to live by thriving!" And you, Bryony Gordon, are one of those brave souls. You and Meghan Markle. So don't for a minute allow Jareth to tell you that you are being self-indulgent for facing your issues head-on. That is *not* self-indulgent. That is the very definition of being selfless, because by dealing with your shit, you get to be more available to your daughter. To your husband. To me.'

'I—'

'I haven't finished. I haven't even got to the bit where you claim that having more than one therapist is excessive. I mean, COME. ON. BRYONY. Have you not won, like, multiple awards for your mental health campaigning? Where is the woman I watched climb up on stage in front of Stephen Fry and Prince

Harry when she was just sixty days sober, the woman who was given a big doorstop of a trophy from Mind for making such a significant difference to the way that mental health was reported in the media? Where is the woman I accompanied to that swish black-tie dinner in London, the woman who stood on a red carpet and was fawned over by a load of mega celebs who thanked her for her writing on OCD and depression and addiction? Where is the woman who crossed the finish line of the London Marathon WEARING NOTHING BUT HER UNDERWEAR? Because I've got to say, I preferred that woman. That woman kicked ass. And I know she's there inside you. I know she still exists. I just think that for some reason – and that reason is probably the enforced isolation of a pandemic – you've forgotten about her.

'Well, let me remind you. She knows that the voice in your head right now, the one telling you that you're being snivelling and self-indulgent, is not your real voice, but the voice of mental illness itself. She knows that it is perfectly fine to have a whole team of doctors behind your brain, in much the same way that it would be perfectly fine to have a whole team of doctors behind you if you had any other chronic health condition. And let me tell you, Bryony, with OCD and addiction, you definitely have a chronic health condition. You have a whole *host* of chronic health conditions, ones that need constant management if they're not going to make your life a misery. It's actually appropriate that you have a team behind you. It's what that woman you've forgotten about has been fighting for all these years: equality between mental and physical health. And proper equality, too, none of this talking-the-talk equality that forgets to walk the walk. Honestly, right now, you sound like some tosspot MP standing up in Parliament to preach about the importance of talking about your mental health, while behind the scenes they're voting to cut funding to mental health services!'

'I think that's a *bit* unfair,' I interject. 'I've only mentioned that I feel slightly silly; I'm not introducing sweeping austerity cuts to public services.'

'But can't you see, Bryony? Every time you give in to the negative chatter in your head, every time you listen to it, you are allowing the stigma to grow. The very stigma you've spent so many years trying to eradicate, so that our kids don't have to grow up in a world where they are called difficult for having an illness that is no fault of their own. Would you be coming to me, telling me that you were being self-indulgent, if you'd been assigned a team by the NHS for a heart condition, or a lung disease, or cancer? Would you be moaning about being self-indulgent if you had to go and see a doctor to fix your broken leg and a physiotherapist afterwards to rehab it? Jesus fucking Christ, Bryony – where has the woman who knows all this gone? Dig deep, find her, and remember that SHE is you, and anyone else is Jareth the fucking Goblin King!'

'That is quite rousing,' I say. 'But actually, I think you'll find that Jareth the Goblin King has been replaced. I can't find him anywhere. I think, maybe, that something has happened to him.'

She sighs. 'And what, exactly, has happened to him?'

'He's been eaten by a new foe that has arrived in my brain. The Stay Puft Marshmallow Man.'

Movie characters from the eighties you could totally name your mental health condition after:

- The Terminator.
- Uncle Buck.
- Hans Gruber from *Die Hard*.
- Freddy Krueger.
- Scarface.
- Beetlejuice.
- Darth Vader.
- General Zod.
- Gordon Gekko.
- Slimer.

6

Ghostbusters

Snapshot from my iPhone's Notes App, January 2021

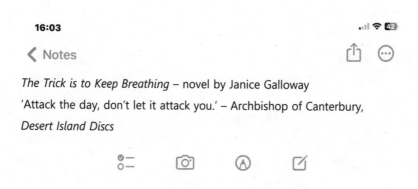

16:03   .ıl 🛜 42

❮ Notes   ⬆️ ⋯

The Trick is to Keep Breathing – novel by Janice Galloway
'Attack the day, don't let it attack you.' – Archbishop of Canterbury,
Desert Island Discs

And so it is that, at the age of forty, with a new fictional character from an eighties movie marauding through my mind, I find myself learning how to eat properly again.

Although, actually, I'm not sure anyone ever taught me this in the first place. Like so many other women my age, I grew up in a culture that taught me to fear food, rather than respect it and see it as something that nourishes my body. A culture where it was perfectly normal for big billboard adverts to shame women for being able to pinch an inch of fat on their hips and belly, where to have even a hint of a stomach was to be called . . . well, the Stay Puft Marshmallow Woman. I remember being given this nickname in year six at school, when my body had had the temerity to grow in line with biology. Tiny buds had bloomed on my chest, buds that would eventually become breasts, and the boys in my class were not going to let me forget it. 'Bryony has BOOBS,' they taunted, as I tried to reach the water fountain in the playground. 'Bryony is BIG. Bryony is THE STAY PUFT MARSHMALLOW WOMAN!'

They roared with laughter at their cleverness. I turned puce and ran into the classroom, horrified by my growing body, rather than the dickheads who had decided to comment on it. Because that was the way back then, that was always the way: it was me that was wrong, not these little boys. It wasn't their demeaning barbs that were at fault – it was me. It was the silver lines on my thighs and my chest, the stretch marks that pronounced me as the witch I so clearly was. And their comments were only the beginning of it, only the start of a lifetime of people who felt entitled to judge the way I looked. From the sixth-form teacher who told me off for showing too much cleavage (I was wearing a perfectly normal vest top), to the men who thought nothing of telling me in passing on the street that they wanted to spunk on my tits, to the online commenters who later in my career saw nothing wrong in condemning my body as a drain on resources. As a woman, there was only one way for me to exist: I needed to be as small as possible, in every conceivable way.

The solution, then, to all of life's problems, was to go on a diet and lose a few pounds. Being bullied at work and unfairly passed over for promotion? Just lose some weight! Husband left you? Just lose some weight! Can't afford to pay your mortgage? Just lose some weight! Need to negotiate world peace? Just lose some weight! The message was not exactly explicit, but it was clear: if you could just be skinny, and smaller, and stop taking up so much fucking space, your life would be a hell of a lot easier for you, and everyone around you.

Genuine things I heard older women say when I was a teenage girl, and never, ever questioned:

- 'We could all do with losing a little bit of weight, Bryony.'
- 'You're too curvy to be a fashion model, but you could be a Page 3 model.'
- 'Those hips will at least be useful when you are pushing out babies.'
- (While pointing to slightly larger woman) 'I don't look like *her*, do I?'

And while I like to think that we've got better at this, I also know that this is bollocks. The only thing we've got better at is making the message more insidious, more creeping, more subtle. Sure, the whole of the internet will kick up a fuss and cancel you if you are stupid enough to promote a product with a billboard that asks if you are 'beach body ready', à la the advert for some weight-loss supplements that was the subject of many complaints in the UK to the Advertising Standards Authority back in 2015, but somehow was not banned.. And sure, you might cause a bit of a fuss if you run a campaign that doesn't include a wide range of body sizes. But if you apologise and then cast a vaguely diverse group of people for your next ad campaign, while still airbrushing them so that there are no lumps, bumps or cellulite in sight, then it will all be quickly forgotten about.

Meanwhile, social media is awash with adverts for crazy weight-loss products that are promoted by the algorithm to anyone who happens to identify as a woman. Filters abound – it is now more normal on social media to look like a photoshopped version of yourself than yourself. To prove this point, an eating disorders charity called the Bulimia Project recently decided to use artificial intelligence to create images of the 'ideal' man and woman according to our use of social media. The results were frightening, though only because it's difficult to tell the difference between the AI renderings and the average contestant on *Love Island*.

According to AI, our ideal human has big hair, big boobs, big muscles, perfect teeth and blemish-free skin. The women are mostly blonde, the men tanned and handsome. None of them are people of colour. All of them pout miserably. Nothing sags, other than your heart as you realise that this is what people aspire to look like right now: computer-generated animations about as human as Mr Potato Head or Buzz Lightyear. Explaining their findings, a spokesperson for the Bulimia Project said: 'We can only assume that the reason AI came up with so many oddly shaped versions of the physiques it found on social media is that these platforms promote unrealistic body types to begin with.'

The truth is that nothing AI produces could ever be weirder than what us humans have conjured up through a combination of filters, plastic surgery and tweakments. Nobody raises an eyebrow anymore at swollen, surgically enhanced lips, or tales of people flying to Turkey to have a butt lift – and not just because their foreheads have been frozen by Botox, which is now as normal as going to the dentist for a check-up.

The messages I receive are not just through the images I see on social media. They are also in the emails and DMs that frequently land in my inbox.

'You suffer from mental health issues because you are fat,' wrote one poor, misguided fool who seemed to have missed the fact that I first got OCD when I was a tiny child, and that my mental health was almost certainly at its worst when I was both bulimic and cocaine-addicted, but also a 'healthy' size ten.

'You are promoting obesity,' emailed someone else, who neatly summed up the strange belief that people can be in partnership with a body type, in much the same way that Michael Jordan is with Nike for sport wear, or Natalie Portman is with Christian Dior for perfume.

All these messages have only ever served to light a fire in my belly: the fire to promote being comfortable in the skin you are in, whatever body shape that happens to be. And yet now, as I begin my work with Naomi, I am realising how deeply ingrained my self-loathing is. And make no mistake, it *is* self-loathing, not 'insecurity', a word that hardly does justice to the emotions so many women feel. And is it really any wonder that we feel these extremes of self-loathing? Growing up, I learned that some foods were good for me but most of them were bad, because they had the ability to make my body undesirable to members of the opposite sex. I learned that to enjoy food was wrong; it was somehow sinful, and not becoming of a young woman. I learned that if I wanted to eat anything more than a Caesar salad, I was a pig. No wonder I also learned to do all my eating in secret.

Indeed, the more I work with Naomi, the more I see how amazing it is that I've had periods of eating normally at all. How amazing it is that I have managed to break through some of the more pernicious elements of diet culture and embrace my larger body in the way I have. That I then went on to run not one but two marathons with it is a tribute to me; I can sort of see that. But it frightens me how easily that work has fallen away in the year since the pandemic began, how quickly I have been reduced to binge eating raw sausages in secret and standing on bathroom scales in an attempt to gain validation. I realise how fragile my mental health still is, how much I will always need to take care of it.

With Naomi, I am essentially reprogramming my brain. I am reprogramming it to learn that bingeing is as detrimental to my mental and physical health as purging, and that when I restrict my food the day after a binge, it only makes me more likely to binge again that evening. I am reprogramming it to remember that it is perfectly normal to eat three meals a day, with two snacks in between. That there are no bad foods. I remember that a whole large pizza is fine, but a whole large pizza plus several bags of crisps is hardly going to leave me feeling on top of the world. I remember that carbs, sugar, fat and salt are simply sustenance, rather than dangerous weapons whose aim is to destroy us.

And I learn things I didn't know before. I learn that eating disorders are so prevalent in part because food is the first way we learn to control our caregivers. When we were weaning as babies, we knew that if we threw our broccoli on the floor or refused a spoon full of pureed potato, we would briefly have some power. I learn that food is so much more than just nutrition. It can be used to influence people, and it can even be used as a weapon during times of war, the providing or withholding of sustenance being just as powerful a tool as a bomb or a gun.

I learn that one in fifty people will experience binge eating disorder (BED), but that only one in four people who live with BED will ever receive treatment for it. I learn that BED is very common in anorexics as they recover from their illness – after long periods in starvation, their brains go into overdrive. I learn that while fasting may be helpful for some people, for many of us who have grown up influenced by a screwed-up diet culture, it is just another way to engage in disordered eating. In 1948, the noted epidemiologist Ancel Keys carried out research that is still known today as 'the Minnesota Starvation Experiment'. He demonstrated that you don't have to be underweight to enter the state of starvation – it can be experienced by anyone with a significant calorie deficit, in a body of any size. The experiment found that after a period of starvation, some participants described feeling anxious and experiencing a 'loss of control' when allowed to eat again. The study found a higher incidence of depression after starvation. This, then, explains the crazy diet culture we live in, and why so many of us seem to 'struggle' with food, yo-yoing endlessly between the states of restriction and bingeing. Turns out it's not the food's fault at all, but the way in which we've been taught to eat it.

But the thing that really strikes me is that recovering from an eating disorder is, weirdly, far harder than recovering from alcoholism. The consequences of my bingeing food might not have affected others in the way that my bingeing alcohol did, but that doesn't make it any easier to stop. And while I don't need to drink alcohol or take cocaine to stay alive (even if, at times, it felt that way), I do have to eat food. Going through treatment is like taking a tiger out for a walk three times a day. It is being thrown to the lions every time you think about breakfast, lunch and dinner. It is running the gauntlet each and every minute of the day, from the moment you wake up to the moment you go to bed, and very often in between, in the form of dreams and nightmares about bingeing.

I experience such nightmares, very occasionally, in relation to booze and drugs. It is usually a vivid and realistic dream where I find myself relapsing, but hiding the relapse, and pretending to everyone that I am still sober. Sometimes, the dream is even worse – it tells me that I have never, actually, been sober at all, that I have quietly continued to drink while maintaining a facade of recovery. I always wake up in a cold sweat from these night-mares, but I find them useful: I see them as my brain's way of reminding me of the dangers of drinking, without me actually having to drink. But the food dreams are revolting. They are like some fucked-up cross between *Charlie and the Chocolate Factory* and *The Human Centipede*: me, rolling in chocolate and cakes and crisps, only for said chocolate and cakes and crisps to start seeping out of every orifice in my body.

One night, Harry wakes me up from one of these dreams.

'You OK?' he asks, propped up on his elbows in the dark. 'You were thrashing and moaning like you were having some sort of night terror, and you're completely soaked in sweat.'

I can feel perspiration between my thighs, under my boobs, on the sheets. I remember the way that, when I was detoxing from alcohol, my body sometimes felt as if it had gone several rounds in the ring with Mike Tyson. Now I am doing a mini detox from crap food. I'm like Renton in *Trainspotting*, only I'm going cold turkey from sausages instead of smack.

I have a sobriety counter on my phone that measures the seconds, minutes, days, weeks, months and years since I last had alcohol or cocaine. Now I add a new counter, which I call 'CHORIZO'. Naomi explains that I can still eat chorizo, I just need to be mindful of it, but it seems to me that just as I need to be completely abstinent from alcohol, I also need to be sober from sausages. There are certain food items that are just like booze and drugs to me. In the words of all great twelve-step fellowships: one is too many, and a thousand is never enough.

'It's like alcohol,' I tell Naomi. 'If you came to me today and told me that scientists had created a pill that would enable me to drink moderately, I wouldn't be interested in it. The idea of only having one or two glasses of wine with my dinner absolutely fucking appals me. I am not interested. I would rather have none than one, seriously. If I'm going to have a drink, then I'm going to have a fucking drink, because otherwise, really, *what is the point?*'

'To enjoy the taste and how it accompanies a meal?' suggests Naomi.

'Don't be ridiculous!' I say, genuinely horrified. 'It may be nearly three and a half years since I last had a drink, but make no mistake, I'm still a raging alcoholic.' And then I tell her about the black-tie awards ceremony I went to at a posh London hotel just before the pandemic, the kind where you are stuck at your table until every single one of the awards for digital marketing and publishing has been handed out, because you've agreed to do the keynote speech after (as if anyone at all in the room wants to do anything other than go outside and smoke a fag at this point).

'So there I am, wedged between a man who wants to talk to me about online engagement insights, and a woman who spends most of her time getting annoyed because there is no signal down here in the ballroom of the posh hotel, which means she can't check her email. And all I can think about is how slowly they are drinking their wine. Tiny little sips, at infrequent intervals. At one point, because I have nothing better to do at a black-tie do now that I no longer drink alcohol, I decide I am going to measure

101

the time he takes between sips. Do you know how long he went at one point? Eleven minutes and forty-five seconds. I repeat: ELEVEN MINUTES AND FORTY-FIVE SECONDS.' I shake my head in disbelief and notice that on my screen, Naomi is looking ever-so-slightly perplexed, like I might be ever-so-slightly mad.

I plough on regardless. 'I wondered if he was drinking so slowly because the waiters had all the booze and were taking their time to come round and refill the glasses. So there he was, telling me more about his online engagement insights, when I just stopped him and asked if he was annoyed. He said, "What about?" And I said, "About the fact that you are not allowed to keep your wine bottles on the table, so you have to wait for someone to come and fill up your glass. It would annoy me, if I still drank, but I don't drink, because I used up my lifetime's drink allowance by the age of thirty-seven, and now I'm not allowed to drink. But if I *was* allowed to, I would find the slowness of the wine refilling, and the general lack of trust that you are capable of looking after your own wine and not drinking it all at once, a little bit annoying. In fact, I'm kind of annoyed *for* you." And he just let out a little laugh and then turned and started talking to the person on his other side, so I guess there was at least one bonus to my observations.'

In truth, by this point, Naomi also looks as if she wishes she had someone else she could talk to.

'All of which is to say, I think it's best I don't go near chorizo for a while,' I sigh. 'I know that no food is bad, and that it's not healthy to start cutting out things from your diet. But in this case, I think I will make a special exception, just until I'm feeling a little less deranged and there's not a global pandemic on anymore.'

Naomi nods, and then changes the subject. 'Can I give you some homework?'

Sign up now for EATING FOR ADDICTS – a revolutionary new course that promises to change your life!

Do you eat your feelings, have late-night chats with your fridge and frequently find bits of crisp in your cleavage? Do you wish you were the kind of person who genuinely enjoys vegetarianism and actively cooks food using lentils?

If so, we have just the programme for you!

Learn how to:

- Eat a balanced meal.
- Take your time while eating, and fully enjoy each bite.
- Stop eating when you are full.
- Open a multipack of Pickled Onion Monster Munch and only have one packet instead of all eight.
- Occasionally leave food on your plate, like those really strange people you sometimes see in a restaurant.

All it takes is a complete rethink of how you live your life, coupled with several months of intensive therapy analysing what has led you to this point. Sign up now before you die of the shame you feel for not being able to eat like a normal human being, despite decades of instruction from the diet culture you grew up around!

The homework is to eat a meal at the kitchen table with my husband, without our phones or any television to distract us.

A simple enough task, you might think, in which case: con-gratulations, you are probably Eckhart Tolle. You are spiritually enlightened and present, and accept that there is only ever now, that this moment is all that matters, and that to dwell on the past or the future or numb yourself from the present is to be unconscious. But I am not Eckhart Tolle, just in case you hadn't noticed. I am not a great spiritual teacher beloved of Oprah Winfrey who believes that if you accept the present moment, you will find a perfection that is deeper than any other form and untouched by time. I am Bryony, a forty-year-old mum-of-one who lives in a falling down house in south London that she is not really allowed to leave all that often because, in a present moment that seems to be going on and on and on and fucking on, there is still a pandemic on that has shut everything down for the second time, just as winter is getting properly started.

Oh, and I am also an alcoholic with binge eating disorder, in case I forgot to mention that.

But even if I was none of these things, I also happen to live in a society utterly dedicated to unconsciousness, as Eckhart Tolle would no doubt say. Everything, and I mean *everything*, is designed to distract us from the great big yawning chasm that exists in each and every one of us. Even Eckhart Tolle. Between social media and streaming services and smartphones, I am not *supposed* to sit at the kitchen table with my husband to eat a meal. I don't even know if we have a kitchen table anymore, so long has it been since we last used it. Instead, we have those little Ikea step stools that, it turns out, make great mini tables for a TV dinner in the living room. Doesn't everyone have these? Surely it can't just be us?

Turns out Naomi doesn't have them. And neither does Peter.

'It's a normal thing to eat dinner at a table with your family,' points out Naomi, as if talking to a small toddler. Which I suppose, in sobriety terms, I am.

'I know that,' I whine, keeping to the role of the small toddler. 'But I just don't see how it helps me with my binge eating.'

'It will help because it will involve you engaging with your food, and your husband, instead of staring blankly at a screen in your hand while the screen in your living room also plays, and you mindlessly put food in your mouth. Because I'm guessing that's what you do, right? It's what most people do nowadays.'

'Well, I mean, I suppose so – yes. And now I come to think about it, we had to stop watching Scandi noir a couple of years ago because we couldn't read the subtitles while also looking at our phones. It was that or learn Swedish.' I laugh, but realise this is not actually that funny. It's kind of tragic that the thought of eating and watching TV without looking at my phone makes me twitch. That the idea of eating without watching any screen at all, while having to engage in conversation, is enough to put me off food altogether.

I think about my relationship with food more generally. Even before this bout of bingeing, I realise it was a little bit strange.

'I don't like going out in the evenings,' I blurt out to Naomi. 'I mean, even before this pandemic. I was kind of relieved when we all got locked down, because it meant I wouldn't have to find reasons to say no to dinner invitations. Eating in public has always made me feel ...' I stare away from the screen and into the middle distance. 'I don't know. Ashamed. Uncomfortable. I've never enjoyed it in the way that I know Harry does. He would love for us to be able to go out to restaurants, or have people round for dinner. I don't think lockdowns have come as that much of a shock to him, because since I've got sober, I've stopped being able to go out properly, so we always just stay in.

'We don't have a social life because I'm kind of scared to have one. And before, I was only really interested in drinking. Now, when it gets to 7pm, I just want to shut down and switch off. It's like the food and the phone and the TV are doing for me what the booze and drugs used to. I go into my own little world, where I'm sort of insulated from all my madness. I get lost in the food, in my phone, so I don't have to sit still with myself. I can see that the way I am is a problem, I really can. I'm just not sure how to solve it.'

'You're not a problem that needs solving,' Naomi says, with real compassion in her voice. 'You're a human who needs to start accepting herself. That's all.'

But I'm not sure I have it in myself to believe her. Not yet, anyway.

I tell Harry that we are going to start eating dinner at the kitchen table.

He looks at me as if I have just suggested we start swinging, or sign up to Feeld as a kink-loving couple looking for a unicorn.

'You what?' he says, when I walk into the study (the spare bedroom) and explain the homework I have been set by Naomi.

'We're going to start eating dinner at the kitchen table, without any screens to distract us,' I repeat, breezily.

'I'm not sure about that,' he says, as if casually dismissing a child who wants him to go and play Barbies. 'It doesn't really sound that fun.'

He turns back to his work. I stand behind him, too stunned to be able to move. After a short while, he realises I am still there and turns back around to look at me. 'Can I help you with anything else?' he asks, somewhat condescendingly.

'Can you *help me with anything else*?' I rearrange my features in a way that I hope gives off 'quizzical emoji face' vibes. 'Let me think about that. I know you've helped me with the alcoholism, and the OCD, and I'm ever so grateful for that, but if you don't mind, I have just one more assignment for you to assist me with, and that's getting over my rampaging binge eating disorder.'

'Oh, right.' He nods. 'The eating dinner at the kitchen table is, like, a therapy thing, rather than a fun thing?'

'You got it!' I give him my most dazzling smile. 'It's homework. It's supposed to help me improve my relationship with food. And you, as a bonus.'

'Oh well, that sounds lovely then,' he trills. 'If you can set the table, I'll make some turkey balls and cauliflower mash. Delicious!'

I smile a rictus grin, and then I go back downstairs to find the kitchen table.

I locate it under the weight of: seventeen takeaway leaflets; a year's worth of water, gas, current account and mortgage statements; several hundred works of art by Edie; three pairs of headphones; £7.89 in loose change; a pencil sharpener; two winter coats; five Ocado plastic bags; some hand cream I have been trying to find for at least half a year; a set of keys of unknown origin; and two terms' worth of home-schooling maths work sheets that were quickly discarded in a sea of tears from both parents and child.

Right, I think to myself, while dumping it all in a bin liner that I will place in the cupboard under the stairs and deal with later. *Let's get to it!*

'What are you doing, Mum?' asks Edie, wandering in from the living room, where she has been creating a massive multi-cultural utopia of LOL Dolls, Sylvanian Families, Lego Friends and Shopkins. 'Why have you put a new table in the kitchen?'

'It's not new, darling.' I wince. 'It's always been there. It's just always been used as more of a . . . storage space, than a table.'

'Cool,' says Edie, putting her head in the kitchen cupboard. 'Is it OK to have some . . . MUM, WHERE HAVE ALL MY HULA HOOPS GONE?'

'Oh, about those.' I begin to make up some sort of excuse, but stop myself, appalled. I realise that the lies of addiction come so easily to me that I often don't even recognise that is what I'm doing.

It is like taking candy from a baby.

Or Hula Hoops from your own child.

7

What the fuck is wrong with you?

Snapshot from my iPhone's Notes App, February 2021

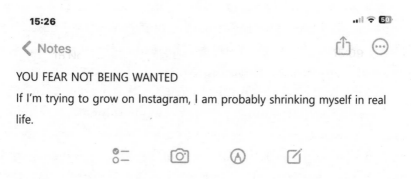

< Notes

YOU FEAR NOT BEING WANTED

If I'm trying to grow on Instagram, I am probably shrinking myself in real life.

If going into combat with Jareth the Goblin King is an exhausting internal struggle, like having the battle for Middle-earth take place in your brain before you've even got out of bed and had a cup of coffee, then taking on the Stay Puft Marshmallow Man is more of a physical fight. I know all too well the *mental* exhaustion of OCD, the fatigue that comes from willing yourself not to get sucked down in endless rumination about intrusive thoughts. But with binge eating disorder, my entire body seems to be in on the proceedings. Every night I go to bed shattered, feeling like a Ghostbuster who has spent the day chasing the Stay Puft Marshmallow Man through the streets of Manhattan with their proton pack. Except I'm trapped in my house in south London, and I don't have a portable ghost vacuum attached to my back in my fight against Stay Puft. Instead, I have regular therapy with Naomi to help me to understand why I binge, and a food diary on my phone.

The food diary is kept in a special app. There's an app for everything nowadays – to order your shopping, to turn down your heating, to tame your rampant eating disorder. This particular app allows me to log everything I eat, so that I can begin to be more aware of what is going into my body. Naomi can see it too, which adds a good dollop of accountability into the mix. The idea is not to punish me, or to make me become (any more) obsessive about what goes into my body, but instead to become conscious of what I am eating. It also means that at the end of each day, I can look back and be proud of having eaten entirely normally.

For some people, eating entirely normally is innate. It is habit. It isn't something they even have to think about. They just open their fridge and reach for a range of healthy ingredients, and then throw them together without giving it a second thought. For them, it is entirely natural to eat nuts, seeds, fruits, vegetables and *lean* protein. 'Oh, this piece of salmon steamed with courgettes, asparagus and fresh herbs?' they say to their millions of Instagram followers, health exuding from every pore. 'I just knocked it up out of leftovers in twenty minutes. It's so easy and delicious and filling!'

For people like me, such a scenario is as fantastical as the idea of Timothée Chalamet walking through the front door and asking for a shag in French. Salmon. Steamed. Courgettes. Timothée Chalamet. Does not compute.

When you are in the grips of an eating disorder, the idea of consuming food in a normal way can feel as overwhelming and unthinkable as the thought of turning down heroin might be for a drug addict. And food absolutely can be a drug, as I am finding out. Highly processed foods, such as pizza, doughnuts and sweets, have been designed to taste delicious, but all that processing means they have more in common with narcotics than natural food, hitting the same dopamine receptors in the brain that a line of cocaine or a glass of wine or a cigarette would ordinarily light up. Some experts have even said that junk food is deliberately designed to be addictive, and that because of this, it should come with the kind of health warnings you see on cigarette packets. All I know is that I finally have an answer as to why I never want to binge on raw vegetables, only highly processed crisps and meat.

The app sends me notifications reminding me to have breakfast, lunch and dinner, and to have snacks in between those meals. By eating regularly, I will feel fuller, and be less likely to binge. If I go longer than two hours without eating, an alert is sent to my phone, to remind me that I need more food. It seems counterintuitive to treat binge eating with more eating, but apparently the idea is to get you back into a regular, non-disordered eating pattern. And yet, at first, my body feels non-compliant. It wants two coffees for breakfast, a snack for lunch, another coffee for an afternoon snack, and all the other meals in one go, somewhere around dinner time. It is, I suppose, the equivalent of being jet-lagged after a long-haul flight – I am binge-lagged after months of disordered eating.

113

When I was in the grip of that disordered eating, I could easily have consumed thousands and thousands of calories in twenty minutes without even realising it. Now I am consuming the same number of calories over the course of an entire day. I can eat whatever I want – no food is banned – I just need to eat appropriate amounts of it. And I don't like it. I find it hard to eat regularly, and 'normally'. As an alcoholic, it's like being asked, every day, to only have two glasses of wine, and leave it at that. I cannot imagine how it would feel to just naturally be like this, to wake up every morning and breeze through the day without giving a second thought to what you put in your body, Timothée Chalamet trying to seduce you in French. What would that be like?

I don't like eating 'normally', but I will do it. I will do it, because I've done this before. I've tackled my problems. I've done it with OCD. I've done it with alcoholism. And I will do it with binge eating. I have to. Because what other choice is there? Letting the Stay Puft Marshmallow Man take over?

As Dan Ackroyd didn't say in Ghostbusters, but really should have done: 'Not today, Gozer. Not today.'

Maybe it's the months of almost exclusively eating processed meat, which can hardly have provided the top-notch nutrition I need to arm me for a daily battle with the Stay Puft Marshmallow Man. Or maybe it's the dark winter days that are really like nights that never end. Or maybe it's the fact that we are only one day into the spring term, and already the government has closed the schools and locked us down again. Whatever the hell it is, I am cream crackered. Completely frazzled. Absolutely spent. I am the melting face emoji in human form, my body collapsing around me in a puddle of shame, self-loathing and 'Next slide, please' broadcasts from Chris Whitty.

Bits of me that are currently on strike until improvements in current working conditions are guaranteed by the person in charge:

- Short-term memory.
- The ability to recall the names of people I have known for years.
- Knees.
- Hips.
- Hamstrings.
- Arch on my left foot.
- Fourth toe on right foot.
- Menstrual cycle.
- Left shoulder.
- The ability to regulate temperature at night and not wake up freezing to death in own sweat.

I want to sleep, all day long. It is a clarion call from deep inside my body. As soon as I am awake, I want to go back to bed, but as soon as I am allowed to go to bed, my body wants to be awake. I am, in the words of one of my late, great, grandmothers, bone tired. I never knew what she meant by this, but now I do. Even my bones want a fucking lie down. They creak with every move, as if they are loudly complaining that they got put in my body instead of one belonging to a Victoria's Secret model. 'Not *this* body!' they whinge, when I stand up after having the gall to sit in the same position for more than five minutes. 'Any body but *this* one!'

My joints, too, are pissed off with me. Pissed off to the point that they seem to have gone on strike. And this is a problem, because I am a keen runner. Not a fast runner – that's a different thing – but a keen runner. And keenness will get you a long way when it comes to running – forty-two kilometres, or 26.2 miles, to be precise. The ability to take off for hours with only my feet for company is one of the things that keeps my mental health on track. Long-distance running as a sixteen-stone woman was not something I ever thought I could do, but then I realised that I had got through multiple episodes of OCD, and if I could do that, then I could totally run a marathon. The discovery that my body was capable of far more than I gave it credit for was genuinely revolutionary for my mental health. It allowed me to see a different path, a different option for living. I could carry on drinking heavily and taking drugs to try and manufacture some sort of temporary buzz, or I could get up and take my body on a fabulous adventure where it can get high all by itself. As a teenager and a woman in my twenties and early thirties, I had always seen exercise as a form of punishment, a way of making my body smaller. But the realisation that I could use it to make my *life* bigger changed my relationship with physical workouts completely. I started to do it not to be fast or strong, but to try and be sane. I started to do it not for how it made me look, but how it made me feel.

I enjoyed, too, smashing through the hackneyed old stereo-types of what a fit person should look like. You know the ones, because, just as I used to, you've probably got them planted in your head. Every time someone found out I had run a marathon, they inevitably asked how long it had taken me to do it. As if they didn't quite believe me. As if they were trying to catch me out and prove that a fat person couldn't actually do exercise.

'What time did you get in the marathon?' they asked, needing desperately to dismiss my efforts.

'What time did YOU get in the marathon?' I would respond.
'Oh, I haven't run one,' they would say.
'Well, there we go. Now, do fuck off.'

The truth is, I have never cared about a time, a pace, or gaining a personal best. For me, it has always been about getting out there and doing it. The endorphin hit I get from forcing myself to go for a run is like no other. And make no mistake – I always have to force myself. I used to have this strange notion that people who exercised sprung out of bed each morning actively *wanting* to go for a run. But soon I realised that nobody *wants* to go for a run. People who do it regularly are simply people who have realised they will never *regret* going for a run. With this lodged firmly at the back of my brain, I have made it a habit, over the last few years, to get out for a run at least three or four times a week.

But now each journey outside feels more like a wade through the gloopiest treacle. My lower back aches, my calves throb, my hips twinge with an intensity that suggests they need replacing. Every time I go to move my leg, or stretch out a quad, my knee tells me to bugger off.

And it's not just the physical stuff; it's the tedium of seeing the same fucking park, day after fucking day. I feel like I know every inch of the duck pond, every blade of grass on the common. It is intensely fucking boring – and it is intensely fucking spoiled of me to be bothered by how boring it is. There are doctors and nurses out there who would give their right arms to be bored right now, and here I am feeling all boo-hoo because I'm currently more inclined than normal to sit on the sofa. I need to pull myself together.

But try as I might, I can't. My body won't listen to the furious missives being barked out by my brain. It is being disobedient, lazy, a complete and utter asshat. It weighs me down to the point that it seems impossible to fight against it. I begin to find reasons not to go out for my regular runs. Excuses, really. I am tired from battling BED all day long. I need to rest. I need to listen to my body. I conveniently forget that often, in the form of Jareth and the Stay Puft Marshmallow Man, my brain will hijack my body and lie to me.

I will go tomorrow, I think, almost every night, without fail. As I lie in bed, I even start to get excited about the run I will do in the morning, how good it will make me feel, the boost it will provide, releasing me from this rut I seem trapped in. But I wake up exhausted, leaden with dread. Maybe today is not the day. Maybe I just need to stretch. And each day, with each missed run, in a teeny, tiny, imperceptible way, I forget the great things I am capable of. I lose a little bit of me.

It's so subtle, so inconspicuous, that I barely even notice it is happening.

In February, it is so cold that the pond in the local park freezes over. My daughter watches the coots ice-skating around, and laughs.

'I wish I could be a duck,' she says, and I know what she means. I wish *I* could be a duck, or, failing that, I wish I could walk on to the ice and have it cave in under my great weight, so I could disappear into the murky black, leaving only a perfect hole on the surface where my body once stood.

The desire to die is immediately engulfed by another desire, to not be such a fucking dickhead. *Pull yourself together*, I think. *You've got nothing to complain about. You have a roof over your head, a loving family, the support of Naomi and Peter, and still you're fantasising about drowning in the pond of a south London park. Jesus! Has it escaped your notice that the hospitals are filling up again? That more and more people are losing their livelihoods? All you have to do is take on a man made of marshmallows, while thousands of people lie in intensive care doing battle with Covid. Why can't you just be content, for once? Why can't you see your privilege, your luck, your immense good fortune? What the fuck is wrong with you, you lumpen piece of shit?*

It's a rhetorical question, of course, but I still have plenty of answers to it. What the fuck is wrong with me, above and beyond the binge eating disorder and the alcoholism and the creaking knees? Let me count the fucking ways.

For a start, I seem to have become incapable of answering phone calls and texts. It's so simple, responding to people. It is the most basic human ability. Even babies can do it, smiling or farting or belching over someone who says 'Coochy-coochy-coo' at them. And yet here I am, forty years of age, completely unable to tap out a response to someone asking how I am, or whether I want to go for a socially distanced walk with them.

I try to reply. I try really hard. I hold my phone in my hand and I stare at it with all the focus at my disposal, and I think about all the many different ways in which I could respond.

• **I could respond like a normal person,** with a breezy, 'Hey, I'm fine thanks, would love to go for a walk, how about in the next couple of weeks?'
 Pros: simple, easy, doesn't take up much time.
 Cons: officially engages the friend in something approaching a conversation. They might reply with a date, or – even worse – a specific time, which would mean I would have to commit to meeting them. Then I would have to spend every waking hour

119

until that point in time I had committed to trying to work out how to get out of said commitment. Could I fake an urgent Zoom call, or a sore throat that might be the new strain of Covid? I could, but then I would feel terrible about lying to them, and I'd worry that they might know I was lying. I would obsess for hours about them thinking I am flaky, and unreliable, and, and . . . Jesus Christ, flaky and unreliable is exactly what I am. So obviously, this line of response is a hard no.

• **I could respond truthfully**, by saying I am fine, but that I have absolutely no interest in going for a socially distanced walk with anyone, anytime soon. I could tell them that the thought of making plans fills me with dread, as does the thought of walking round the same park having the same conversation about Boris Johnson for the 462nd time this year.

    Pros: honest.

    Cons: a trifle blunt.

• **I could not respond at all**, instead becoming distracted by some sort of home-schooling/work dilemma and forgetting about the message entirely until three weeks later, when I wake in the middle of the night in a cold sweat feeling terrible guilt for my rudeness.

    Pros: probably the most popular way of dealing with WhatsApp messages these days.

    Cons: gets a bit tedious after a while.

My WhatsApp inbox makes me feel like a Minion trying its very hardest to do an impression of a human. Try as I might to be a responsible adult, I just can't. I find interacting with other people harder and more exhausting than any marathon I have run. The truth is, I don't want to go for a socially distanced walk with anyone. I have no chat, no small talk, no jokes. It has taken me so much willpower just to summon the energy to read the message, or listen to the voice note, that I have nothing left inside me to actually go for a walk. And speaking of voice notes . . . just, *why*? 'Are you checking in, or launching your new podcast?' I want to scream into my microphone, but I don't, because I'm too busy. Being misanthropic.

All over social media, people are posting about how much they miss their friends. But I don't miss my friends. I don't miss them, and I *really* don't want to see them. Don't get me wrong; I like my friends. Some of them, I even love. But I have absolutely no desire to be anywhere near them. To be anywhere near *anyone*, actually, other than my husband and daughter. I don't pine for social gatherings, for the opportunity to be *out*. I pine only for the opportunity to be *in* – inside my home, inside my shell, inside what I believe to be the safe cocoon of my head. I have even come to dread invitations to Zoom parties, which are like real parties, only without the canapés. And when you're an alcoholic who isn't allowed to drink, the whole *point* of going to parties is the canapés.

Then there's the fact that I have started going to bed at 7pm. At first, I thought my extremely early nights were a simple matter of circadian rhythms – when it gets dark at 3pm, I really can't see the problem with crawling into bed a few hours later. But at some point, I realise that other adults my age – and by 'other adults my age', I mean my husband – don't go to bed at 7pm. They don't eat dinner with their seven-year-old, and then have a bath with her, and then read her a story and switch off the lights at 7.05pm, as if this were a perfectly normal way for a forty-year-old with a mortgage and responsibilities to behave.

'Maybe we could stay up tonight, sit at the kitchen table, try doing some of that homework again?' suggests Harry one morning, like the absolute sociopath he is.

'Oh, perhaps we could go to the Moulin Rouge for a bit of a dance while we're at it.' I know sarcasm is the lowest form of wit, but really, what does he take me for? Someone with energy?

I try to explain the exhaustion to him, but fail, on account of being too tired. It's like there's a button between my eyes and the button gets switched off every day at around ... well, 1pm. If I'm lucky. On particularly bad days, it never gets switched on at all. Some people wake up to an alarm clock. Others to their child climbing on them. I wake up to the sound of what remains of my brain attempting to clunk back to life.

I wish I wasn't an addict, because if I wasn't an addict, then I would be able to take diazepam. Then again, if I wasn't an addict, I probably wouldn't be craving diazepam in the first place. It's hard to know, really, given the landscape of things. I'm sure there are plenty of people who would like to knock themselves out and wake up when it's all over. All I know for sure is that there are many, many people out there who have it far, far worse than I do, and that I really need to pull myself together.

But instead, I welcome the sun – or what exists of the sun – setting at 3pm. I welcome the darkness setting in, because it means I can surrender. I can give up the fight against the day. I can switch off the lights, and myself, and give up for another twelve hours. It's so much easier than staying awake, trying to face the darkness of the night without booze or food or drugs.

Fantasies in my forties

- Being hospitalised with exhaustion.
- Winning a trolley dash at Sephora/Space NK.
- Getting a Nando's discount card.
- Having a utility room.
- Knowing another language without having to actually learn another language.
- Becoming best friends with Dawn French.
- Winning *Strictly Come Dancing*.
- Being able to sing showtunes.
- Never having to shave my legs/armpits or do my bikini line ever again.

And then, every morning, I realise my mouth is in shreds. Great big sores have appeared in every crevice. My jaw aches. My tongue moves round and feels the indents where my teeth have clamped down, causing the tender tissue of the inside of my mouth to swell and sometimes break. There are toothmarks along the side of my tongue, perfect moulds of my molars pressed into my flesh. It is as if, deprived of my binges, I have started trying to eat myself. I buy a mouthguard.

It keeps me awake.

Within weeks, I have bitten through it.

I am irritable, cranky, half dead behind the eyes.

'Do you think you're depressed?' asks Harry one day.

'Who *isn't* depressed?' I snap. 'There's a pandemic going on! How else are we supposed to feel? Over the fucking moon?'

'I'm just wondering if there's anything we need to do, that's all.'

'Anything above and beyond the two therapists I have, the

twelve-step support group I attend, and the strongest dose of antidepressants known to man, woman or elephant that I take?'

He sighs. 'I'm just checking in, that's all.'

I feel bad for being so thoughtless. There are people out there right now who are lonely and isolated and would do anything to have this kind of connection.

'Sorry,' I murmur. 'I'm just tired. Thank you for doing that. But I'm fine. Absolutely fine.'

8

I think I might be dying (part 698)

Snapshot from my iPhone's Notes App, July 2021

❮ Notes   ⬆️ ⋯

Invite list for forty-first birthday party (really postponed fortieth birthday party)

- Harry
- Edie
- Mum and dad?
- ?????

　　　　　　　☰　　📷　　Ⓐ　　✐

127

15:00

〈 Notes

Things we could do

- dinner?
- horse-riding (Edie's idea)
- arcade at Southside Shopping Centre (also Edie's idea)

The summer of 2021 arrives, and things begin to open up again. Social lives restart. The sun comes out. I go on holiday and pretend to be a normal person for a couple of weeks. I pose for pictures in my bikini and post them on Instagram, and the likes perk me up, like a line of cocaine, only more wholesome. 'I would rather have cellulite on my thighs than hate in my heart!' I write, and it's true. But the problem is, I don't seem to have *anything* in my heart, other than a vague feeling of dread.

The Stay Puft Marshmallow Man seems to have receded into the shadows, beaten there in part by Naomi and therapy, but also by my ferocious fear that binge eating might somehow lead to binge drinking. In recovery, people speak often about 'relapse drift', a term that explains how gradual the movement from abstinence to drinking and using can be. A relapse might seem sudden, but there are many experts who believe that really, they happen slowly, over time, and long before you've actually picked up a drink. As a result, some therapists get you to keep a list of things to watch out for, things that might be a sign you are drifting towards a relapse: not going to twelve-step meetings, hanging around with people who drink heavily, that kind of thing. And though I rarely find myself thinking about alcohol anymore,

I know that the way I have recently been thinking about food is not really any different.

I have to take this stuff seriously, for the sake of my sobriety. Because without my sobriety, I am nothing. Worse than that, without my sobriety, I *have* nothing. My family, my friends, my career, every single thing that I value in life: if I pick up a drink, it all vanishes in an instant.

So, like any self-respecting sober woman in their forties, I do what I have to do.

I take up cold-water swimming.

Things to remember when taking up cold-water swimming

- Wetsuits are for wimps.
- Always acclimatise – do *not* go for your first swim on New Year's Day unless you want to make yourself very miserable.
- Get out wanting more.
- When you start to feel you could stay in forever, that's actually your body going into hypothermic shock.

You're welcome.

Tooting Bec Lido is just a couple of hundred yards from the A214, and yet when I walk through the gates and past the trees that protect it from the rest of the world, I feel a million miles away. OK, so it's not the Caribbean. The water is too cold, and the sound of the trains rattling between East Croydon and Clapham

Junction is too loud, but the point is, it's not my bedroom. It's not my head. If my head *were* a public leisure facility, it would be more like the manky indoor pool round the corner from me, where the showers don't work, the floors are covered in matted hair and discarded plasters, and the air temperature always seems to be a suffocatingly humid thirty-five degrees (the water's still freezing, somehow).

No, in contrast to this, Tooting Bec Lido is a slice of heaven. If it were a human, it would be Harry Styles. It is all multi-coloured Victorian bathing huts, and turquoise-blue water. The people are as cool as the temperature of the pool; they cycle over on big, pastel Pashley bikes, jump into the water without giving it a second thought, swim a mile in sub-zero temperatures, then change into their work clothes under a dryrobe without a) looking like a wanker, or b) flashing their bums.

I am completely out of my depth, naturally.

Without even realising, I mark myself out as a clueless interloper in several ways. Firstly, I buy the bright pink and camo dryrobe – you know the one – which is more expensive than a winter coat from, I dunno, Balenciaga. (I've never bought a winter coat from anywhere other than Uniqlo, so may be making this up.) Later, I will learn that the bright pink and camo dryrobe is seen as the dryrobe for wannabes who are more interested in posting pictures of themselves on Instagram than they are in experiencing the many benefits of cold-water immersion. If you want to appear serious, it is far better to opt for the navy blue one, or even better, a dryrobe that isn't actually made by dryrobe, but by a far smaller, independent company that you found on Etsy and who make their non-dryrobe dry robes at their kitchen tables from recycled bum bags, or something.

Secondly, I turn up without a swimming cap, labouring under

the mistaken belief that the only point of them is to keep your hair dry. And because I am beyond caring if my hair gets wet or not, but not beyond caring if I look like a condom on the world's most flaccid penis, I decide not to spend the extra £15 on a swimming cap. This, despite having spent close to two hundred quid on a coat that looks like a sleeping bag for Second Lieutenant Barbie.

But it turns out that a swimming cap has precious little to do with keeping your hair dry. Silly, vain me! Turns out it's to keep your hair out of your face when you are swimming a ferocious front crawl (which I'm not), and to keep you warm when immersing yourself in water so cold that you have to have a diagnosed mental health issue to even begin considering getting in it outside of the one hot day of the summer.

I may not have a swimming cap, but I do have a diagnosed mental health issue – three or four, actually – which is perhaps why I find myself plunging into Tooting Bec Lido on a misty morning in late October. I let out a scream the moment my toes break the surface, which is the next way in which I mark myself out as a newcomer: it's not the done thing to shriek or complain about the cold this early in the winter swimming season. In October, the water is still hovering somewhere around fifteen degrees, which is practically balmy when compared to what it can get down to (sometimes, they have to break the ice to let the swimmers in, I am told).

It's also not the done thing to spend longer getting into the water than you spend actually swimming in it.

Twenty minutes forcing myself down the steps.

Ten minutes swimming.

And while ten minutes doesn't sound like very long, it turns out it *is* too long if you've been fannying around in the cold for ages beforehand. Which is how I end up making my next schoolgirl error: whimpering inside the changing cubicle as I realise that jeans are the last thing you want to try and put on when you are still partly damp and standing on wet concrete in south London in late October.

'Are you OK?' comes a friendly female voice in the cubicle next to me.

'I'm great!' I call, shivering, trying to put my left leg into my knickers without falling over into a puddle of my own making.

And for that moment, at least, it's true.

I buy a swimming cap, switch out jeans for tracksuit bottoms, and decide to give up on bras (my fingers are too cold after a swim to fasten them back up, and you can't see how perky or otherwise my boobs are under the massively oversized dry-robe). As autumn turns to proper winter, I catch the cold-water swimming bug, like the complete cliché I am. But I don't care if it makes me look like a middle-class stereotype. It is one of the few times in my day I feel truly awake, and it gives me a purpose: that purpose being to swim through an entire winter in only my swimming costume and cap (and beanie hat, should it get particularly chilly).

Day by day, the temperature drops a tiny bit, and my respect for my body rises. Its ability to tolerate colder and colder conditions amazes me: thirteen degrees, twelve, eleven, ten, and down and down it goes, winter's progress bringing with it some of that long-lost appreciation for my body that, pre-pandemic, had powered me through marathons half-naked. Each morning, I arrive at the lido feeling creaky, and a little bit fearful about the day ahead. And each morning, I leave feeling completely unstoppable.

If a *little* nippy.

But by the afternoon, the exhaustion has set back in, deeper even than before. Once I am home and at my laptop, I have a maximum of four hours of work in me before the shutters start to come down. I can set a timer by it. I work ferociously for those four hours, barely stopping for breath. I do not go to the loo, or get snacks, or look at my phone. All that matters is I get as much done as I can before the lights go out in my brain for another day. I am lucky that I have worked from home since before the pandemic; I do not know how I would explain this to my boss if I had to be in an office every day. Would I have to lock myself in a loo for power naps? And how is it that less than a decade ago, I regularly used to be able to function at work on no sleep after an all-night bender? I have no desire to go back to the days of cocaine binges, but what I would give for even a smidgen of the energy I used to be able to summon after those long, crazy nights.

It is a tiredness quite unlike anything I have ever experienced before: deep, treacly, all-encompassing. Nothing I do holds it off. It is no match for caffeine, for cigarettes, for any other legal stimulant that I am allowed to rely on without breaking my sobriety. By 2pm, I am pulled under by it. I set an alarm for 3.15pm so I don't forget to pick up my daughter from school; then, I spend the rest of the day feeling dry-mouthed and lazy. I do not understand how people wake up at 7am and then keep their eyes open all day until 11pm. It is simply incomprehensible to me, like the idea of climbing Everest or speaking fluent French back to sexy, seductive Timothée Chalamet.

My brain keeps going blank, mid-sentence. Mid-thought. Mid-word, sometimes. My short-term memory is shot to pieces. I may not be drinking alcohol anymore, but sometimes I feel as if I am emerging from a million little blackouts each day. I cannot remember what I did three hours ago, let alone last week. I can recall conversations, but not who they were with. I finish a book, and immediately forget what happened in it. I walk into rooms and have no idea why I am there; I open web pages and find myself staring at the Google logo, wondering what it is I am looking for. My brain? My point? A new dress from Zara?

I make the mistake of mentioning this to an editor I work with from time to time. Another Zoom meeting, another hour where I find it hard to concentrate on any conversation because of the sight of my great big moon face staring back at me. Despite knowing exactly where it is, I am unable to click the button that removes my face from the screen. It isn't that I like looking at myself, more that I like being able to see how my chins are creasing under my face at any given moment. I know this isn't normal, to be looking at your own pixelated reflection all the time, but it feels like some twisted form of control during a period when I have very little. By looking at that little box, I am able to watch myself perform for an audience. For a few moments each day, I can imagine I am not a woman in her early forties who has recently waged an imaginary battle in her head with a character from Ghostbusters, but instead a slick talking head on a documentary about . . . I dunno, David Bowie.

The editor is a man, about fifteen years older than me. He is stylish, I suppose, in the way that many men in their late fifties believe themselves to be stylish, having bought a pair of glasses that make them look like a sort of John Lewis version of Jeff Goldblum. We are supposed to be talking about a writing project, but because we haven't seen each other since 2019, we, of course, have to devote the first fifteen minutes of our hour-long meeting to making crap jokes about Zoom and lockdowns and Matt Hancock. Every time someone makes a joke about Matt Hancock, a part of me wants to tell them that it's OK, we don't have to do this. We can skip this part where we poke fun at former cabinet ministers and instead just move straight to rage-filled screaming and weeping. But I don't, because maybe it's just safer to laugh along and even crack a few funnies myself – 'Gosh, I can't wait to be in a room with someone I haven't married or given birth to!' is my standard line at this point of the pandemic – before expressing gratitude for the roof over my head, the air in my lungs, the food in my fridge, while pointing out that others have it far worse, and so on and so forth.

The editor makes a joke about Chris Whitty, which I appreciate, if only because it's not about Matt Hancock. Then I ask him how he is.

'Truthfully?' He smiles, his teeth ghostly white.

'Truthfully.' I nod, wanting to encourage an atmosphere of vulnerability, because it's a hell of a lot more interesting than an atmosphere of small talk, or an atmosphere of faux-cheeriness.

'OK, well, here goes.' He turns his face away from the screen, and for a moment I think he is going to start crying. Then his eyes are lighting up, his mouth twisting into a smile, his head shaking uncontrollably in mirth. He is *laughing*. 'Truth is, things have never been better, Bryony.'

I smile at him and hope I don't look too surprised.

'I feel bad saying it,' he says, though his body language suggests he doesn't feel bad at all, 'but the pandemic has been the best thing that has ever happened to me.'

'Wow!' I say.

'I know, right? Like, my relationship with my wife and kids is so much better. We suddenly had all this time together, and we realised how much we'd missed it. How much we'd needed it. We've really thrived with this new way of working flexibly.

And I know that it seems weird, given we are in the midst of the greatest public health crisis of our lives.'

'Hopefully coming out of it!' I interrupt.

'But I've never felt healthier, mentally *and* physically.'

He closes his eyes as if even he can't believe it.

'That's so great.' I wince.

'My wife and I really went on a health kick when the first lockdown happened. It was like, this awful thing is happening and there are people who are really sick. How can we take this terrible thing and turn it into something good? So we decided we needed to start valuing our health. I thought of you, Bryony, giving up alcohol and getting clean, and I was really inspired, you know? Like, if it wasn't for people like you, I could have very easily spent that first lockdown in a dark place.'

'Oh,' I say, slightly stunned.

'I mean, I know you already run loads and do lots of exercise and obviously don't drink, so what I'm saying won't be anything new to you, but to my wife and I, valuing our health became something really important in that first lockdown. We quit booze, went vegan, ordered weights on Amazon, signed up for an online workout programme. It really changed our lives. And now we just have so much energy. Way more than we did when we first got together in our twenties. And that's just, you know, kick-started everything for us. I feel so much clearer mentally, I have so much more enthusiasm, and so work is really going well. It's all just ... *vibing*.'

'Vibing,' I repeat, as if it might catch on.

'I've decided now that I only want to hang with other people who are on this frequency, you know?'

'I do know,' I lie.

'How about you?' he asks.

'Truthfully?'

'Truthfully.' He nods.

'I'm fucking exhausted. I wake up most days and want to go straight back to sleep. My lower back really hurts, and I think my knees have given up the ghost, so I haven't run properly without stopping at least every ninety seconds for a good year now. I have to have grandma sleeps every afternoon for an hour because otherwise I can't get through the day to 7pm. I didn't go vegan during the first lockdown, largely because I managed to develop something called binge eating disorder, which mostly involved ingesting very large quantities of raw cooking chorizo in the dead of night. On the plus side, I've taken up cold-water swimming, though that's only because six-degree water is the sole place on the planet that my brain feels alert enough to remember my own name. Oh, and I've started having these mad flutters in my chest that come on completely randomly when I'm sitting down doing nothing.' I look at him and smile. 'Other than that, it's been absolutely fucking brilliant.'

We move quickly on to proper work chat, but for some reason, the project never quite gets off the ground.

Search engine

Q Wh . . .

Q Why do I have so much chin hair suddenly?

Q When will I get my period again?

Q Where has my confidence gone?

Q What is wrong with me?

The flutters in my chest are something I have been trying to ignore for a couple of months now, a bit like all chat about new Covid variants, or Matt Hancock's sex life. If I just stick my fingers in my ears and refuse to listen, they'll go away, right?

I think these flutters are palpitations. Or stress. They don't seem to be a heart attack, on account of the fact I am still alive, but obviously I have consulted Dr Google just to be on the safe side. My search history is littered with questions and statements like: 'flutters in my chest, am I dying?'; 'exhaustion, memory loss, insomnia, pain in right arm, should I call 999?'; 'signs I am having a heart attack'; 'woman early forties overweight occasional smoker chances of heart disease?'

I am self-aware enough to know that if you spend a good portion of your day googling the symptoms of physical illnesses, the chances are you're probably suffering from a mental one. For me, health anxiety is the number-one indicator that my brain needs a good rest. It's a sign that Jareth is on his way. One minute, my brain is saying: 'Are you absolutely *sure* you don't have terminal cancer, or AIDS, or that you're not having a heart attack or a stroke?' The next, it's telling me I am the worst person since Fred West. For me, it's just a short hop, skip and a jump from hypochondria to stressing that I might be the next Adolf Hitler.

I also know that the signs of a panic attack – clammy hands, racing heart, shortness of breath – are exactly the same as those of a heart attack. You don't work in mental health campaigning without being able to diagnose panic disorder in someone. So, for a while, I nestle vaguely uncomfortably in the knowledge that this is probably what is happening to me. I'm just having occasional panic attacks. If I go to the doctor about this, they'll pat me patronisingly on the head and thank me for wasting their time.

But as the end of 2021 approaches, the occasional flutters in my chest start to feel more like the pounding wings of a ptero-dactyl. I am sitting at my desk one day when the pounding strikes up out of nowhere. It's as if my heart is trying to break free from the arteries that have it trapped in my body. It has joined my bones and joints in an all-out protest at having to exist inside me. It is trying to pump its way out of my chest. It is throwing itself aorta-first at the flesh and muscle that separate it from fresh air. And speaking of fresh air, I desperately need some. I am light-headed. I cannot move. My vision narrows to the single point in front of me, which happens to be the middle of my laptop screen, which right now is displaying an article about Kim Kardashian's bum, as I try to write a piece about the tyranny of shapewear. I try to breathe in through my nose, but I am scared that might hasten my heart's escape. My jaw aches. My arms ache. My back aches. I am dying, and I am certain of it, and when they find me, they will think that my heart gave out over the excitement of Kim Kardashian's arse.

Somehow, I manage to lie down on the floor, under my chair, away from the sight of anyone's bottom. I put my hands on my chest and feel my heart thudding erratically inside it – flopping around with no rhythm or regularity, like the almost-dead thing it is. I remember I have an Apple Watch, and that it tells you your heart rate. I look at my wrist, and see that my heart is beating at 187 beats per minute.

It doesn't even pump at that rate when I'm running.

I want to call for help, but there is nobody in the house, and anyway, I don't have the energy to make any noise. So I lie there, breathing deeply, willing my heart rate to go down. A few minutes pass, and I do not die. The thudding seems to stop. My heart rate becomes very, very slow, like it has almost used up its daily allocation of beats and now has to ration them for the rest of the day. I go to stand up, and quickly realise that this is a bad idea. My head is still woozy, and I don't think my legs will support me.

When I am eventually able to sit up, I know that even if this is just a panic attack, it's probably better to get a medical professional to confirm it for me, rather than relying on Dr Google. Exhausted, unable to hang on even to 2pm, I grab my phone, crawl into bed, and text Harry to tell him he needs to pick Edie up from her playdate, because I am not feeling well. Then I call the doctor, make an appointment, and fall asleep until the next morning.

The doctor tells me I need to lose weight.

They always do this.

'Have you thought about taking up exercise?' he asks me, staring directly at his screen. 'Even some light walking might make all the difference to you.'

'I *do* exercise,' I snap, irritably. 'I've run two marathons in the last five years.'

'Oh really?' he says, his interest piqued. 'What was your time?'

'I can show you the medals if you want,' I say, 'but I'd rather discuss the possibility of doing some, I don't know, tests or something? Because it was quite worrying, the episode the other day.'

'I'm sure it was, Ms Gordon.' He smiles patronisingly. 'I'm happy to order some blood tests to reassure you that everything is OK, but in the meantime, I really think you could benefit from losing a few pounds.'

He hands me a pamphlet about healthy eating, and sends me on my way. Outside, I throw the leaflet in the bin, light a cigarette, and try to swallow back the hard ball of emotion that seems to have formed in my throat.

Things weight loss MIGHT help with:

- Diabetes.
- The risk of heart disease, stroke and some cancers.
- The desire to wear a smaller dress size.
- A lack of respect from your doctor and other people who have very binary views about health.

Things weight loss WON'T help with:

- Your intrinsic value as a human being.

A week later, I see the letters 'GP' flash up on my phone. I am in the Apple Store in Covent Garden, getting the E, R and T keys on my laptop replaced. I excuse myself from the Genius, who has been polite enough not to ask if I use my fingers to type, or small hammers.

'Hello?' I say into my iPhone.

'Oh, Ms Gordon?' It is the doctor, presumably calling to ask if I've lost any weight, or if I've managed to get together any proof that I actually ran those marathons I told him about.

'Yes.' I try not to groan.

'It's Dr M—— here. I'm calling because we have the results of your blood tests, and while most of them are perfectly normal, there is something I *am* a bit concerned about that I think we need to look into.'

'Oh,' I say, noticing that the Genius has her septum pierced as well as her eyebrow, but not her ears.

'Yes, you have quite a high platelet count in your blood,' he says.

141

'Right,' I say, admiring the tattoo of a lion's head on the Genius's wrist.

'And a high platelet count can be a sign of cancer, I'm afraid.'

'Really?' I respond a little breezily. '*That's* interesting!'

'So what I need you to do is go to the hospital within the next few days to have a chest X-ray and a mammogram, just to check it's not lung or breast cancer. We will send a stool test kit to your home which will enable us to rule out bowel cancer. I can get the practice nurse to text over all the information about where to go for the other investigations. Have you got any questions?'

'Am I going to die?'

'We're all going to die, Ms Gordon,' he says. 'We're just going to send you for some tests to make sure it doesn't happen anytime soon, OK?'

'OK,' I repeat. 'Well thanks for letting me know.'

I hang up, and walk back to the Genius, who has finished fixing my keyboard.

'All OK?' she says, handing me back my laptop.

'All fine,' I smile. 'Absolutely *fine*.'

9

Relapse

Snapshot from my iPhone's Notes App, December 2021

< Notes

Stay alive

Try to go out in the evening without suffering paralysing anxiety for weeks beforehand

Move to wilds of Cornwall

Start a commune

All the tests take place in the hospital where I had my daughter eight and a half years earlier.

I sit in a plastic chair waiting for a chest X-ray, and think about that version of me: what a child she was. What a naive, foolish juvenile. I think about how she worried about such seemingly petty, trifling things: breast or bottle; Bugaboo or Baby Jogger; baby-led weaning or pureed broccoli and beans. This version of myself is as distant and strange to me as the version of myself who sat on a beach in Thailand less than two years ago with a bunch of LOL Dolls, wanting to celebrate the beginning of a new decade. A new decade that has, so far, brought with it only misery and suffering and isolation and – less importantly, though quite crucially for me – a mushroom cloud of self-doubt that at times makes me wonder if I'm about to evaporate into thin air.

It wouldn't be true to say that I am scared as I sit in the plastic chair waiting for the chest X-ray – more that I am astounded that I have managed to stay alive long enough to arrive at the point of sitting in this plastic chair waiting for a chest X-ray. It genuinely baffles me that there have been points where I have just cruised through life without realising how absolutely useless I am. Without realising what a liability I am. How have I existed without the basic level of self-awareness that is necessary for most people to function? I feel a hot shame in my stomach, a sense that for my whole life, people have been noticing what I have been incapable of seeing: the absolute pointlessness of me. The sheer fucking arrogance of my clueless fucking existence. How dare I have left this hospital eight and a half years ago, toting a baby in a car seat, assuming that I would be able to parent and adult and not immediately fall into an alcoholic stupor, picking up exactly where I'd left off before I got pregnant?

146

As I wait to be called in, I realise that this particular visit to the hospital is clearly a case of karma. It is punishment for all the many mistakes I made after the birth of my daughter. Being at the pub and drunk within two weeks, and back on drugs within six weeks. Not sobering up until she was four. Modelling addiction and disordered eating to her, and having absolutely fuck all decorum by then *writing* about said experiences in newspaper articles and books that people actually read. This brush with *genuine* health issues, not silly cosseted ones in my brain, is clearly my penance for being so self-indulgent.

Things people feel entitled to email and tell me:

- That I am fat.
- That I am fat and Jewish.
- That I am self-obsessed.
- That I am a drain on the NHS.
- That I am a bad mother.
- That I should be sacked.
- That they feel sorry for my husband.
- That they'd like to sexually assault me.

'Bryony Gordon,' says a man in scrubs, clutching a clipboard. Or at least, I think that is what he says from behind his mask. I rise from my seat and make my way towards him, smiling broadly, even though a) I too am wearing a mask, so he won't be able to see said smile, and b) I am not here to make friends with him. Why am I like this? Why is it that everywhere I go, I need to make sure that nobody mistakes me for a difficult

147

woman? What would happen if, even for a fleeting moment, the man in scrubs *did* think I was a difficult woman? Would he refuse to X-ray my chest and throw me out of the hospital in disgrace? Or would he be more likely to find terrible things on my X-ray, the terrible things being retribution for being a difficult woman?

He sends me to a changing area that is a bit like a fitting room, except that instead of waiting to find out if you have discovered the golden unicorn that is a Zara dress that actually goes over your head, you are waiting to learn if you have lung cancer. A woman hands me a blue gown. She tells me to remove my bra and my top and my jumper and put the gown on, and then to go and find the man in scrubs, who will be waiting for me in room three. I do as I am told, keen not to be seen as anything other than biddable and compliant. My boobs hang pendulously under the fabric of the gown, like udders on a cow.

In room three, the man in scrubs hunches behind a computer screen. He doesn't say hello as I walk in, or ask how I might be feeling; he just instructs me to stand in front of a great big box that will scan my chest for evidence of the terrible things that will be there as punishment for being a difficult woman. I'm paraphrasing – obviously, he doesn't mention terrible things or how bothersome I may or may not be.

I stand in front of the big box and wonder if he is horrified by the sagginess of my tits. Then I wonder why it is that I care. I decide to crack a joke as he presses various buttons, and a series of lights and sounds whirr around me, like the world's shittest disco. By cracking a joke, I realise that I am behaving like someone trying to break the ice on a date. 'Can you tell that I used to smoke twenty Marly Lights a day in my twenties, forty on a night out?' I wince at my use of the term

'Marly Lights', but also at his silence in the face of my 'joke', which, I realise, in the context of a radiology department, is not that funny.

Eventually, he asks why I am here, in a tone that suggests I am wasting his time.

'Why am I here?' I repeat, surprised by this line of questioning.

'Yes, why did your GP send you here?' He has the demeanour of a man who has been rudely interrupted, like my grandfather when I used to ask him to play snap while he was watching the horse racing.

'Because I had some weird blood-test results that he said needed looking at more closely.'

'Yes, I can see that, but the numbers are barely high enough to warrant further testing.'

'I wouldn't know about that,' I say. 'I'm just doing what I have been told to do.'

'OK, well, I'll write to your GP with my findings. You're done.'

I stand with my boobs around my waist, wondering if my nipples are visible through the gown.

I want to say: 'Sorry, but when you say "You're done," do you mean that in a "You're done, everything's fine and you can go home" kind of way, or a "You're done and your time here on this earth is coming to an end because your chest X-ray shows evidence that you are about to shuffle off this mortal coil" kind of way?'

But I think that might make me seem a bit difficult, so instead I say: 'Is there anything on there that I should worry about?'

He seems to let out an involuntary snort, as if I have asked him the world's stupidest question. 'I can't see anything worrying. I'll need to take a closer look, but I've got no reason to keep you here for any more tests.'

He motions towards the door. I am so relieved by what he has said that I forget to be angry about all the difficult *men* I have encountered in the medical profession in the last two weeks.

The nurse carrying out the mammogram is gentler, even if the same cannot be said for the equipment that squashes my boobs into fleshy pancakes. She, too, is not concerned by what she finds – or doesn't find – in my breasts. Thankfully, nobody is present when I have to provide a sample of my shit. That comes back smelling of roses, too.

'Your tests are all clear,' says the GP when he calls me two weeks later.

'So what caused those unusual blood-test results? And why did I have that funny turn with the palpitations?'

'The high platelet count could have been caused by any number of benign reasons. You might have had a virus that raised it. It's hard to know for sure. What matters is that we've ruled out any of the more *sinister* causes. As for the palpitations,' he says, his voice becoming deeply patronising, 'they were probably caused by stress. I can have some information sent over to you on breathing exercises and mindfulness, if that might help? Also, do think about losing some weight.'

'Fuck off, I know how to breathe,' is what I want to say, but conscious of not being difficult, 'No thank you,' is what falls out of my mouth instead.

'OK, well, is there anything else I can help you with?' I know he doesn't mean that, that he has about thirty seconds remaining before he has to terminate this call and move on to the next one.

'I just want to check that there's nothing I need to worry about,' I say, seeking reassurance.

150

'You're fine,' he says. 'Absolutely fine.'

There's that word again.

On 24 February 2022, the government removes all pandemic restrictions, and yet I am in the midst of a lockdown far more prohibitive than any I have experienced in the previous two years.

The type I got pretty used to, once upon a time.

The type that I thought I had banished when I got sober.

The type that involves being locked inside my own head, rather than my own home.

I can't say for sure when I start to doubt what I see before me, but I think it is at some point in January, shortly after I test positive for Covid for the first time. It's a routine test, the type required by a venue to make sure I am safe to come and do a talk about mental health. On the morning of the event, I wake up feeling fine – and by 'fine', I obviously mean 'no more awful than usual'. I am tired, but when *aren't* I tired these days? It would be more of an anomaly, at this stage, to feel alert and perky. I sit on my bed and remove the packaging of the Covid test the venue has sent me. I go through the motions, like the former drug-addicted bulimic I am: no squeamishness *here* about shoving things up my nose and down my throat. My eyes water a bit, but nothing out of the ordinary. I swish the swab in the vial of fluid, pour the fluid on to the lateral flow cartridge, and go to the bathroom to have a shower. I am so convinced of my invincibility that it isn't until I have my hair dried and my make-up on that I bother to look at the result: two clear lines that automatically stop all plans in their tracks.

I should be disappointed, but I am delighted. I am delighted because it means that for the next five days at the very least, I have

151

a legitimate reason to isolate from the rest of the world. No talk tonight, no walks tomorrow, no making and then breaking plans to go for coffee. I am blissfully free to not have to leave my house.

I post a picture of the two lines on my Instagram stories to alert people to the fact I will be AWOL for the foreseeable, am surprised by the number of people who reply congratulating me on my pregnancy, and then call my husband to tell him the good news.

'I have Covid!' I rejoice.

'Oh, thank fuck for that,' he sighs. 'I just saw your Instagram story and thought you were calling to tell me we were having another baby.'

'Don't worry, there's no way I am actively choosing to have another child with someone who still doesn't know what a lateral flow test looks like.'

'I can see that you're not so ill that you have lost your ability to be scathing.'

'I'm fine, just weirdly relieved that I don't have to go and do this talk tonight. I was feeling . . .' I go quiet for a moment, and realise I was feeling *panic* at the thought of having to talk to other humans, of having to interact with them and socialise with them and just generally be around them. 'I was feeling anxious that I might be coming down with something and that I would give it to everyone. I'm glad I know for sure now.'

I don't even realise I am lying.

I just think I am speaking a more bearable truth.

Because the actual truth?

I'm still not ready to see it.

On the fourth day of testing positive for Covid, I am so congested with phlegm, so unable to sleep, that Harry goes to the chemist and buys me some medicine. I gratefully receive it, think of how pleasant its sharp tang is, and conk out for fifteen hours.

On the fifth and sixth and seventh days, I take the medicine again, because it is like getting under a big, fluffy duvet and shutting out the world, and when you are delirious, veering wildly between fever and cold sweats, that's about the only place on the planet you can cope with.

On the eighth day, feeling slightly better, I look at the medicine, and realise it has a small amount of alcohol in it. Horrified, I put it in the wastepaper bin in my bedroom.

That night, feverish once more and again full of phlegm, I go and retrieve the bottle of medicine, and take a small spoonful to help me sleep.

Then I put it back in the wastepaper bin.

On the ninth day, I wake up with an appalling voice running through my head.

'You have relapsed,' it says.

'You have broken your sobriety,' it taunts.

'You are *bad*,' it repeats, again and again and again. 'You couldn't just deal with the Covid, sweat it out, as a properly sober person would. You took a drink, in the form of the cold and flu relief medicine. You basically went *bin-raiding* for booze. You need to reset your sobriety date. You need to go to the next available twelve-step meeting and announce you have relapsed and that you are a newcomer. You need to go back to the beginning and restart the steps.'

I begin searching sobriety forums, seeking some sort of reassurance against the voice in my head. Surely, this can't constitute a relapse? Surely, I'm being super paranoid? I find a query from another sober person who has experienced something similar to me, and read with horror the responses.

'WHY ARE YOU MESSING AROUND WITH YOUR PRE-CIOUS SOBRIETY?' queries one person.

'The fact you even need to ask suggests to me that you know the answer,' says someone else. 'I just don't understand how, after all the hard work you have done getting sober and going to rehab, you would risk it by taking medicine with alcohol in it. Like, I don't even have mouthwash. It's just not worth it for me.'

I feel sick. Relapsing is literally my worst nightmare – one I have frequently – come true. I google how much alcohol is in the medicine I took, and am relieved to see that even if I was to drink the whole bottle in one go – which I didn't – it would be the equivalent of a very small glass of wine. A relapse, then, or a slip? I call Holly, shaking.

'I think I've relapsed,' I splutter to her, in tears.

'Wait, what?' She sounds confused. 'I thought you were at home with Covid. How have you relapsed?'

'I took medicine that had alcohol in it, even after knowing it had alcohol in it.'

'OK,' she says, calmly. 'Bryony, did you drink the whole bottle or something? Because if you did, you probably need to go to hospital and get your stomach pumped for paracetamol.'

'No, no, I just had the correct dosage,' I say, though that voice in my head cautions me that I can't be sure; that I might have somehow got my hands on another bottle and drunk it, and that I might now be dying of an overdose.

'OK, well, if that's the case, why do you think you've relapsed?'

'Because I knew it had alcohol in it, and yet I still took it. Can't you see? I need to reset my sobriety date!'

'Bryony, I think what you need to do is take a deep breath. Are you at home? Is Harry with you?'

'He's at work, Edie's at school. Holly, I can't believe I've relapsed. I can't believe I've fucked it all up.'

'Bryony, I don't think you've relapsed. I think you've been sick and had some medicine, and you're not feeling great.'

'But I didn't really *need* the medicine, did I? I mean, it wasn't as if I was really, really sick, like all those poor people who have had Covid and ended up on ventilators, or died from it. I just had a fever and a cough and was bunged up; I could have got through it without medicine. I feel like I've failed.'

'Have you had an actual proper drink, Bryony?'

'No! No, of course not! The thought of a drink horrifies me!'

'OK, so only you can truly say if you've relapsed. It's the intention, not the substance. Like, did you take the medicine because you were sick, or because you wanted the alcohol?'

'Because I was sick,' I say, because it's true, it really is. 'But I've still had alcohol. And don't we always say in twelve-step meetings that alcoholism is "cunning, baffling and powerful"? What if this is it being exactly that? What if my brain is telling me I took it because I was sick, when actually I took it because I wanted alcohol? Shouldn't I reset my sobriety date? I feel like if I don't, I'm being dishonest. I need to tell everyone what has happened so that they don't think I'm something I'm not, so that they know how fraudulent I am.'

'Bryony, my love,' says Holly, as kindly as possible. 'I don't think you need to do that. I think what you need to do is take a moment, ground yourself, and then make an appointment to see Peter.'

'He's going to be so cross with me,' I say, starting to sob.

155

'Oh, Bryony,' replies Holly, and I think I can hear a crack in her voice too. 'He won't be cross with you. Sweet, lovely girl, *nobody* is cross with you.'

But that's not true. Because I am. I'm cross with me.

10

Shame

Some people feel shame and hide it deep inside them, a secret that seeps into their bloodstream and starts to poison their whole body. But I am so used to shame that I can no longer bear it; I cannot keep it in me for a moment longer than it needs to be there. I feel the need to expunge it, to clear it from my body by confessing to it. If I can admit to it, and seek reassurance, then it will go away, right?

Over the next few days, unable to leave the house, I call other people in recovery, other alcoholics, and I treat them like priests in a confession booth. I go through every detail of my 'relapse', every thought and action that might have led to it. I run through all the ways in which I am bad, all the ways in which someone stronger and better than me would have resisted the cough medicine and seen out the Covid through ... I don't know, prayer? Meditation? They listen, patiently, because that is what people in twelve-step fellowships do. They listen, and they do not judge. They have been there. They have sinned, too, and someone has sat patiently with them as they have confessed to those sins.

Harry thinks I am behaving in a deranged manner. He thinks that it is nuts that I am putting myself through the wringer over some cough medicine. He says that when I was drinking and using, before I got sober, cough medicine was the least of my worries. He reminds me that I used to go AWOL for days, that I would find myself in crack dens with strangers doing drugs and putting myself in danger.

But he doesn't get it.

I may not have been doing cocaine, or downing tequila, but who is to say that this won't happen if I don't catch the alcoholism early and correct its course? Who is to say that the cough medicine wouldn't have led to coke binges if I hadn't stopped it in its tracks? He thinks that I am safe because it's been almost five years since I went on a bender, but he doesn't realise that alcoholism lives inside me, doing pull-ups, waiting patiently for the day that it can sneak back in and take over.

I need to be vigilant. I need to be on guard. I need to hold myself accountable for my actions and not get complacent, because if that happens, all hell will break loose. I can't afford to err. I can't stray. I can't be bad. I can't, I can't. I just *can't*.

Peter, when I eventually test negative and am able to see him, is quite clearly horrified.

Not by the cough medicine, but by how absolutely *mental* I seem to have become in the three and a bit weeks since I last had therapy.

He doesn't say this, of course. He wouldn't be allowed to, but nor does he actually need to. I can see it in his face, as I sit and tell him what has happened, about the cough medicine, and needing to reset my sobriety date, and how absolutely terribly I have behaved. As I speak, he tilts his head in that curious way of his, like a labrador wondering why you would be so strange as to hold a ball and not throw it. His right eyebrow is slightly cocked, as if he is having trouble computing the information I am telling him, his mouth half ajar. He waits for me to finish speaking, and then I take a deep breath in expectation of his judgement.

'It sounds like you've had a tough time.' He speaks softly, *without* judgement, and I can't bear it. I want him to flagellate me, to flay me, to sentence me to a life of suffering. I want him to tell me that I have relapsed, that I have fallen back into active addiction, that I am bad, and irresponsible, and that I have let down my husband and my daughter, but most of all myself. I want him to tell me that I can't let *him* down, that he is merely disappointed in me, that he had never allowed himself to get attached enough to feel anything stronger, because I mean so little to him, and always have; it makes no bones to him whether I live or die, but I should know as well that it's been a long time since he has had a patient who is quite so hopeless, quite so self-pitying and pathetic. I want him to tell me that I am so despicable that he can no longer have me as a client, and furthermore, that he will let it be known to other psychotherapists that it would be unwise to take me on, so futile a case am I. I want to pay him to do all of these things. I will pay him double, treble, whatever he wants, if he will just spit on me and tell me what a useless piece of shit I am.

Instead, after a long pause, he says this:

'Bryony, I am really, really sorry that you have been in such pain these last few weeks. I am really sorry that you have suffered like this. I wish you had reached out or got in touch, because I can see how awful all of this must have been for you. How awful it still is for you. That's the first thing I need you to know.'

There is a pause. The tears prick my eyeballs and start dripping down my face.

'The next thing I need you to know,' he continues, 'is that you *have* relapsed, but not in the way you think you have. You don't need to reset your sobriety date, or go to a twelve-step meeting and announce you are newcomer again. You don't need to restart the steps, unless that's something you *want* to do. You don't need to do any of this, because you haven't relapsed into alcoholism, Bryony.'

My throat begins to ache as he speaks; my chest starts to heave. It's like I know what he is about to say.

'The thing you've relapsed into is OCD.'

And there it is. There *he* is, the figure I thought I had managed to banish, the one I thought had disappeared. He's there, sitting on the sofa next to me, laughing, because really he has been there all along.

Jareth. Jareth the fucking Goblin King.

Some of the many different things that OCD can make you question obsessively:

- Whether you might hurt someone.
- If you really love your other half.
- Your sexuality.
- Whether or not you are good enough.
- Whether you might be a serial-killing paedophile.
- Whether you might have accidentally taken an overdose or put bleach in your drink (or someone else's).
- Real events that have actually happened, and whether you have remembered them correctly.
- Whether thinking about something bad happening will actually *make* something bad happen.

- Whether you've balanced out the bad thoughts with enough good thoughts.
- That you might have sent someone an abusive message and then deleted it without realising.
- That you might be a racist.
- That you might have been assaulted without realising it, or have assaulted someone without realising it.
- Whether or not you have a sexually transmitted disease.
- The safety of absolutely anything that is precious to you, including but not limited to: your children, your partner, and your sobriety.

You'd think that finally being able to see Jareth would make him easier to catch. That after months and months and possibly years of waiting for him to turn up again, his presence right in front of me would make it easier to swing a net over his stupid bouffant hair and capture him, before locking him away for all eternity and throwing away the key. But here's the thing: Jareth is as cunning and as baffling and as powerful as alcoholism, if not more so. He is a shape shifter, a form thrower. When I was twelve, he made me question if I had AIDS; at thirty-five, he made me wonder if I was a serial-killing paedophile; and now, at forty-one, he is making me doubt whether I am really sober. He attaches himself to anything you value dearly – your home, your family, your career, your sobriety – and he sets about destroying that thing while also convincing you that you are actually protecting it. Because as you obsessively ruminate and check your behaviour, you disconnect entirely from all that matters. You lose your ability to live and love and laugh and do anything other than exist in the clutches of his compulsions. You fall under his spell without even realising that is what is happening.

Jareth the Goblin King has inveigled his way back into my brain. He's crept in quietly, with stealth, over the course of the pandemic. I can see that now. I can see him, his stupid fucking peroxide-blond Status Quo hair and his ridiculous fucking tight trousers and his absolutely ludicrous crystal ball-topped sceptre. I mean, it would be laughable if it wasn't so *obvious*. He's been there all along! All that worry that I wasn't worried enough about Covid; all that obsessing about good and bad and right and wrong ... that was *Jareth*! It was just Jareth, dressed up as Chris Whitty!

Even the Stay Puft Marshmallow Man ... even *he* was one of Jareth's attack dogs. Or attack marshmallows. Binge eating disorder was just another way of making me feel bad and wrong and faulty, like the alcoholism and the bulimia and every other fucking negative thing about me. It's all been Jareth, the *whole time*.

'Of course it's been me,' sneers Jareth from my frontal lobe, where I see he has set up a luxurious purple velvet chaise longue in front of a roaring fire. I look around, see the extent of the home he has made in my head: the walk-in wardrobe full of silk shirts, the cupboards full of Jim Henson puppets.

My whole brain, I realise with horror, belongs to him.

Every morning, I wake up and forget for a moment.

For five blissful seconds, I come round and I am a normal person in a normal house with a normal life. I am free, unencumbered, good to go.

Then Jareth wakes up too and has a very strong cup of coffee. Not one of those weak-arse filter coffees that hotels give you at buffet breakfasts to save money; one of those seriously potent robust blends with an intensity of fourteen that is the closest legal substance to cocaine.

164

'Good morning!' he trills into my ear, like the absolute fucking psychopath he is.

'Fuck off, Jareth,' I weep.

'I love it when you talk dirty to me.'

'Go away!' I cry. 'Leave me alone!'

'Sorry,' he says, not really sorry at all. 'This is *my* brain now.'

And so it is.

February turns to March. People shake off their masks and their bubbles and their need to socially distance, and they return to something approaching normality. They make plans for holidays. They socialise. They says things like, '2022 is going to be *the* year!' and I think, *Oh my fucking god, how has this happened? How has a fictional character from a 1980s movie come to be in charge of my mind in the Year of our Lord 2022, when I thought I had seen him off for good some time ago?*

There are facts that are true, that are impossible to refute. I am forty-one. I am married, with a child and a mortgage and a job. But then there are the things that Jareth fills my head with that make me wonder where he ends and I begin. The things he tells me are horrifying, awful, and yet they are also persuasive and convincing; I know I shouldn't believe that I am the bad person he tells me I am, but if I ignore him, am I only proving him right?

I once described OCD as your brain refusing to believe what your eyes can see: that the oven is off, that the hair straighteners are unplugged, that your hands are clean, that the bump you went over in the road was a speed bump and not a child. Now I realise that it is also like having an entire chorus of extremely convincing conspiracy theorists in your head, who question every single thought that so much as enters your brain, analysing and

165

deconstructing each word, searching for a meaning that doesn't necessarily exist.

As the spring of 2022 becomes lighter, my obsessions and compulsions become darker. I move from worrying I might have relapsed to worrying I might be a serial-killing paedophile. It's always this way with OCD – one minute you're checking your hands are clean, the next you are in an existential crisis about whether or not you have the capacity to commit murder. From morning until night, Jareth and his army of deranged conspiracy theorists chatter away, seemingly without any need for loo breaks or to stop and have lunch. Don't they at least want to go on a five-minute break to get a snack? Apparently not. It is exhausting, dispiriting and entirely demoralising. It is like living with your own personal version of an alt-right news channel in your brain, one dedicated entirely to all your potential fuck-ups and failures. Let's call it 'BG News', for simplicity.

BG News

BG news anchor, who, in my head, looks a lot like Nigel Farage: This evening on BG News, we will be discovering all the secrets about Bryony that she doesn't want you to know. From relapses to serial killing, you're going to hear it here, first.

Co-anchor, who my tormented mind conjures up as Jacob Rees-Mogg: That's right. If you thought Bryony was a respectable writer and mental health campaigner, then I'm afraid what we are going to tell you this evening might come as a shock.

Nigel: But as a fearless news channel dedicated to showing you the reality of the mainstream media – or MSM, as we like to

166

call it – we know we have a duty to deliver you the truth, no matter how uncomfortable it might be.

Jacob: Tonight, we hear from a whistle-blower who has bravely come forward to reveal the full extent of Gordon's depravity. Having lived with her for over three decades, our guest this evening knows the journalist better than most. Now, for the first time, he's talking about what really goes on in her head.

Camera pans out to man who looks a lot like David Bowie, wearing a frilly shirt, waistcoat, jodhpurs and knee-high boots.

Nigel: Jareth the Goblin King, thank you so much for joining us tonight. We know how hard it must have been to come here, especially in trousers that tight. Can we start by asking why, after all this time, you have decided to expose Gordon?

Jareth: Well, I'd like to start by saying that you remind me of the babe.

Nigel *(looking confused)*: What babe?

Jareth: The babe with the power, of course.

Jacob: What power? I love power!

Jareth: The power of voodoo.

Nigel: Who do?

Jareth: You do.

Jacob: Do what?

Jareth: Remind me of the babe.

Stunned silence

Nigel: Right. Anyway. If we could perhaps get back to why you are here?

Jareth: Of course. Well, I should explain that right from the beginning, I asked for very little from Bryony. Just that she feared me, loved me, did as I said . . .

Nigel: Sounds reasonable.

Jareth: And then I would be her slave.

Jacob nods.

Jareth: If she had only been a little more *accommodating*. *She* asked *me* to move in, don't forget. When she was twelve and her hormones started – well, she needed my presence in her frontal lobe to ensure that she wouldn't err from the chosen course, which is, of course, to be good. I only wanted to make her feel better, to make sure she was extra vigilant about all the many dangers out there in the big bad world. If she could say with 100 per cent certainty that she was a good girl, a really, really good girl, then life would be much easier for her. You see, don't you?

Nigel and Jacob nod.

Jareth *(juggling some crystal balls)*: But I'm afraid that from the moment I moved in to her frontal lobe, she was difficult. She questioned my authority, if you see what I mean. I would have moved the stars for her, and yet she started to get uncomfortable when I made the perfectly reasonable suggestion that she wash her hands every two minutes to protect her from germs. I mean, you will remember that back in the early nineties, AIDS was rife, and I didn't want her to fall prey to such a terrible, shameful illness.

Nigel: Well, quite!

Jareth: Her mother had a baby when Bryony was twelve, and obviously I needed her to be able to say with absolute certainty that she would never harm the baby. But I'm afraid, gentlemen, that I witnessed her having *actual thoughts* about throwing her brother on the floor. And that's just the stuff I can say on a respectable show such as yours. No matter that she appeared to be appalled and tormented by these thoughts, I had to know for sure that she wouldn't act on them. So I would lock her inside her head for a good few hours a day, rebroadcasting those dark thoughts to her almost permanently to make sure that there was no positive feedback when they went through her brain, only horror.

Jacob: That was very selfless of you, Mr Goblin King.

Jareth: Please, just call me Jareth. Anyway, as she got older, and she was exposed to more adult situations – sex, alcohol, drugs, and so on and so forth – things only got worse. I would make sure that she spent a good proportion of the day ruminating on the sexually intrusive thoughts that popped into her head unbidden, to make sure she wasn't going to act on them, but then in the evening, in an attempt to dampen the thoughts or get rid of them, she would drink vast amounts of alcohol, well above the safe level for a woman, and then she would also take illegal narcotics so that she could continue to drink alcohol.

Jacob: That is truly shocking, Mr Goblin King.

Jareth: As I said, you can call me Jareth.

Jacob: Mr Goblin King, I insist. Tell me, while she was behaving in this frankly *unladylike* manner, carousing and the like, how did that make you *feel?*

Jareth: Well as you can imagine, intensely worried for her morality. And yet, when I tried to talk to her about it, she used all sorts of colourful language that I am afraid bordered on the abusive. On many occasions, she told me to go fuck myself with a *carrot*.

Jacob *(to the camera)*: We do apologise for the fruity language used.

Nigel: More vegetable-ey, really.

Jacob: Well yes.

Jareth: But it gives you an idea of what I was up against.

Nigel: Tell me, why didn't you leave?

Jareth: How could I? I was trapped in her brain, a labyrinth of immoral thoughts. Without me, she might have acted on them. Then, when I discovered she was pregnant, obviously I really had to step into action to protect both her and the baby. And as for the 'father', I felt she really needed to be able to provide me with iron-clad evidence that he *was* the father. Because what if she was leading an innocent man along and telling him he was the dad of this unborn child, when for all I know, it could have been a stranger she met on a night out and drunkenly had sex with down a dark alley? And yes, you *may* think, well, surely a woman would remember such a moment in her life, but we aren't talking about *any* woman here, we're talking about one who has a history of alcohol and drug abuse, and who would use that alcohol and those drugs to sedate me. She couldn't be trusted.

Nigel: Good grief.

Jareth: Once we had established that the father *was* who she said it was, I obviously had to protect her in other ways. Could she be *absolutely* certain that her baby was breathing all through the night? Could she know for sure that she had sterilised the baby's bottle thoroughly? What if some random germs fell on the baby's bottle and made the baby sick? What if she accidentally put bleach in the bottle instead of formula milk? And isn't formula essentially bleach? I mean, you might wonder why a woman wasn't feeding her baby with breast milk, and obviously that was something I had to take up with her. Because if she didn't care enough about her child to make breastfeeding work, who is to say that she wouldn't harm the child in any other way?

Jacob: Speaking as someone with 800 children, I really applaud the safeguarding practices you were putting in there. But tell me, did she appreciate them?

Jareth: Sadly, no. She kept asking me to leave her alone. In the evening, once the child was asleep, she would drink alcohol again to try and silence me. But the thing about trying to silence someone like me is that the next day, I will shout even louder. I will *not* be silenced.

Nigel: Tell us, what is it about her behaviour recently that has made you want to speak out?

Jareth: Well, gentlemen, it's hard to explain, really. After thirty years, I thought I had seen it all. Then the pandemic hit, and I couldn't believe that after everything I had tried to teach her over the decades, she still didn't get it.

Jacob: Can you be explicit about what you mean by that, for anyone at home who isn't au fait with this level of non-compliance?

Jareth: She wouldn't be a good girl. She knew what was expected of her: stay home, save lives. And yet still, she couldn't do that without complaining. She was a healthy woman while people out there were dying, and yet she disrespected the dead by taking to binge eating. Consuming grotesque amounts of fatty, toxic food. Even when the world was in a state of crisis, the likes of which had not been seen since the Second World War, she couldn't comply. She couldn't quietly do what she was told, without causing any trouble. She had to make it about *her*. She had to be *bad*.

Nigel: It really is quite unbelievable.

Jareth: But there's worse, Nigel – far worse. Having got sober, one of the few good things she ever did in her life, she put it all in danger by taking cough medicine that contained alcohol. *Alcohol*, I tell you. At which point, I had to really kick up a fuss, because if she relapsed, she would surely destroy not just herself but everyone around her. So I had to start asking really

171

tough questions: Are you sure that glass contains water and not gin? What if you took a swig from your husband's beer bottle when he wasn't looking? Should you really be using hand sanitiser that contains alcohol? What if you accidentally got a bit in your mouth? What would happen then? Do you think it's honest of you to be going to AA meetings and claiming to be sober? Don't you think you should be a little more transparent, given recovery is supposed to be all about truth? And speaking of truth, and alcohol, now seems as good a time as any to revisit some of the evenings towards the end of your drinking and using, when you brought strangers into your home while your child slept peacefully upstairs. But how can you be sure she slept peacefully? How can you know, given your extremely altered state, that you didn't harm her on one of those nights out? That one of the strangers didn't harm her?

Oh, she seems perfectly happy now, but can you really be sure that she isn't terribly damaged by your behaviour in active addiction? Can you say with 100 per cent certainty that you didn't harm your child while you were drinking and using? Should you really be allowed to *have* a child? Do you even know what it means to be a mother? Shouldn't you go to the police and tell them how you behaved, and then let your husband and daughter get on with their lives without you? Don't you think that, given all of this, you need to give back any of the success you have accidentally accrued, the awards and the book deals and the columns and the friends? Give them all back and apologise for ever having accepted them? And when I said all of this, you wouldn't believe it, but she started *crying*.

Nigel and Jacob roll their eyes in unison.

Jareth: Weeping, as if she was the *victim*. As if she wasn't the perpetrator. At that point, I knew I needed to go public.

Jacob: If you knew Bryony was watching, what would you say to her?

Jareth *(turning directly to camera)*: I would say, Bryony, you are a fraud. You are tiresome. You are annoying. Nobody wants to know about your stupid issues anymore. You are too much, and not enough, all at the same time. You are terrible. You hurt people, not just with your words and your actions, but with *your very existence*.

Nigel: Thank you, Jareth, for your bravery, not just in coming on the show tonight, but also in living with this monster for so very long, and protecting us from her.

Jacob: After the break, Nadine Dorries and Katie Hopkins will join us to discuss how best to be a good girl. See you soon.

Welcome, people, to my brain in March 2022.

11

Davina McCall

Snapshot from my iPhone's Notes App, March 2022

‹ Notes   ⬆️ ⋯

Ten 10ks in ten days challenge

PURPOSE: to show that exercise is for everyone and raise money for Mental Health Mates

PEOPLE YOU NEED TO BEG TO JOIN YOU ON YOUR ADVENTURE:
Fearne Cotton (good excuse to hang out); Adele Roberts (inspirational!); Paralympian David Weir (also inspirational!); Dr Amit Patel and his guide dog Kika (cute!); Mental Health Mates walk leaders from around the country (legends!)

Incredible as it may seem, I am able to get up and take my child to school and be a parent and have conversations with people I bump into in the street and write pieces for publication in a national newspaper. I also complete a challenge that involves running ten ten-kilometre runs in ten days, to raise money for the not-for-profit organisation that I accidentally set up in 2016, because heaven forbid I sit still and face my own problems before trying to fix everybody else's. Even more absurdly, I genuinely believe that I appear normal as I do all these things, that I am indistinguishable from the pre-pandemic version of myself, who wore £150 bikinis made from recycled fishing nets and read *The Road Less Travelled* for shits and giggles. That nobody can *tell*.

I get up every morning and I look at my hairbrush and think, *Not today, Gozer*. Then I go to the bathroom and, as I sit on the loo, I think about having a shower – but really, what's the point, given that the people I spend most of my time with are Jareth, Nigel and Jacob, who seem to be broadcasting 24/7 on both BG News and Fuckwittery FM? I brush my teeth because I am wracked with enough self-loathing to not want to offend anyone with bad breath, but if you think I'm going anywhere near make-up or an iron or smart clothing, you must be crazy.

'Bryony,' says Holly, when she eventually manages to drag me outside to a twelve-step meeting. 'Do we need to talk? Like, *properly* talk?'

We are standing outside a building in south London, and I am drinking my fourth coffee of the day. It is nine thirty in the morning. My hair is still wet from the lido and I am wearing my bright pink and camo dryrobe. I think I am doing a good impression of a fully functioning forty-one-year-old: cold-water swimming, lots of coffee and an AA meeting, all before 10am on a Saturday! I think I am absolutely fucking *winning*.

'We can properly talk if you want,' I say, lighting another cigarette. 'But I don't know if there's all that much to report.'

'Mate, you know I care as little as you about appearances. But you do look completely *exhausted*.'

'That's because I got up early and went for a bracing swim and, if you must know, I'm having a bit of trouble sleeping.'

'Are you OK?' she asks, moving away from the smoke coming out of my cigarette. 'You are sucking pretty furiously on that fag.'

'I'm fine.'

'Oh my god, you used the word fine! Things must be really bad.'

'What do you mean? I *am* fine.' I throw the cigarette on the ground, crush it under my shoe, and start rummaging for the packet of Marlboro Gold in the pocket of my dryrobe.

'No, Bryony, you are not fine. Come on, you were the one who taught me this! If you were fine, you wouldn't use the word fine. You'd say, "I'm good, thanks" or "Really well!" But you wouldn't say "fine". Only people who are not fine say they are fine, as a sort of polite way to say, "Please don't ask me any more questions about my wellbeing, as I am not in the mood to probe any deeper with you."'

I move my face into a look of surrender, then light another cigarette, my third in five minutes.

'OK, you got me.' I inhale, exhale. 'I'm not fine. The OCD is on me pretty bad. I'm hoping nobody notices, but in truth I keep expecting someone to come in and forcibly remove me from proceedings. To lock me up and throw away the key.' I realise a big tear has splodged down from my face and extinguished my cigarette. 'The truth is, I would welcome being locked up. Just to get a break from all of this.' I motion around my head and my messy hair, and realise I must look a little like the dog in the *What-a-Mess* books I used to read with my sister in the mid-eighties.

'Coffee,' says Holly, linking her arm through mine and walking us away from the building. 'Or a decaf coffee for you. Maybe even a camomile tea. And definitely no more cigarettes, because I'm scared you're going to develop emphysema by 11am. Let's go.'

In the cafe, there are cinnamon buns and custard tarts and they are playing Whitney Houston, so I immediately feel much better.

'Tell me what is going on in that magnificent head of yours.' Holly puts her arm around me, and I feel her shoulders physically drop as she bites into a pastel de nata.

'Oh, you know.' I sigh.

'I don't know, though. I don't have OCD. Tell me.'

'Honestly, if I went into it, I'd just end up freaking both of us out. It's like ... look out there.' I point out the window at the clear blue sky, at the hint of spring in the trees. 'It doesn't matter that the sun is shining and the blossom has started to bloom. To me, the world just gives off a generally dark, apocalyptic feeling. Like the end is nigh. I don't think it's felt this bad since I got sober. And I kind of thought sobriety would cushion me from it ever getting this bad again. Like, if I wasn't putting alcohol and drugs in my body, then, without the chemicals coursing through my veins, I wouldn't sink quite as low. And I know that's ridiculous, because when I first experienced OCD I was only about twelve, and the hardest drug I'd done was Calpol. But I thought that being in my forties, and with all the fucking work I've done on myself, I might be able to see an episode coming.' I lean my head on Holly's shoulder. 'But this one has completely blind-sided me.'

'How are your periods?'

'My periods?' I sit up and look at Holly with what I imagine is extreme bemusement. 'That's a bit of a random question, isn't it?'

'Nope. I'm just listening to you and thinking that maybe you're peri-menopausal. I mean, you are in your forties now. I've been reading loads about it, and apparently mental health issues are a massive sign that your hormones are up the spout.'

I roll my eyes. 'I would dearly love to be able to explain away what's going on with the menopause. It would be terribly con-venient given how trendy it's be—'

'Bryony,' Holly interjects, sternly. 'The menopause is not a *trend*. It's a biological process that fifty-one per cent of the popu-lation can expect to go through.'

'OK, that was bad of me, especially as part of said fifty-one per cent. What I meant was, the menopause doesn't explain my madness from the age of twelve through to thirty-five. At what point am I going to stop looking for a cause for my seemingly never-ending problems? If I had a pound for every time a stranger emailed me or messaged me on Instagram to tell me they think I have ADHD or bipolar disorder or some other condition that they are absolutely not qualified to diagnose in me, I would be very rich indeed. Certainly able to afford to pay for the best therapists in the world to sort out whatever the problem *is* with my head. But isn't it time I just accepted the truth?'

'What's that?'

'That I'm a bit of a fuckwit. That I am fundamentally faulty. There's nothing wrong with me, above and beyond the fact that I'm one of life's great dickheads.'

Holly spits out her mint tea. '"One of life's great dickheads"! Move over Sigmund Freud, we have a new psychotherapeutic genius in town!'

'But it's true! And anyway, let's just say, for argument's sake, that I *am* menopausal. I fear that even the Davina McCall treatment isn't going to help me in my quest to stop worrying that I'm a serial-killing paedophile. Also, my periods are fine, thanks. Lovely and heavy and *gushing*.'

'Bryony, I can confidently say that you're not a serial-killing paedophile.' Holly sighs. 'But I'm afraid I can't reassure you that you're not completely and utterly disgusting.'

'Gushy, gushy, gushy,' I sing, before stealing a bite of her custard tart.

I go home and spend a few hours googling the perimenopause. I think that at forty-one, I am too young to be experiencing it. But it turns out this is as deluded as believing I look a bit like Kate Winslet if you squint while peering at me from a certain angle, or that I might one day win *Strictly Come Dancing*.

While the menopause usually happens in your early to mid-fifties, I learn that the perimenopause can begin at least a decade before, and sometimes in women in their thirties. I scour the endless list of symptoms, and think that they read like a sort of laundry list of my life. Mood changes, trouble concentrating, heavy sweating ... I mean, who *hasn't* been experiencing these since they were about twelve? I check off symptom after symptom in disbelief. Heart palpitations! Difficulty sleeping! Feeling tired or lacking in energy! Feeling dizzy or faint! Sore gums! Needing to wee more often! Loss of interest in sex! Feeling unhappy! Loss of confidence! Reduced self-esteem! Brain fog! It's like taking part in a really crap quiz, where the prize for taking part is learning that any minute now, you're probably going to start experiencing bladder problems and vaginal dryness.

I had thought that menopause involved a few hot flushes and

the end of periods. But now I realise that it is essentially a Tough Mudder, without the medal or finisher's T-shirt. As I read article after article, a familiar rage begins to bloom inside me: the rage of a woman remembering that her lot in life is to just put up with this shit.

Conversations with my mother: Part two

I call my mum, because surely she understands the injustice of your genitals shrivelling up and your bones going on strike the moment that you turn forty?

But she just wants to tell me what she and Kelly from Waitrose have been discussing at their bi-weekly coffee mornings.

'Mum, do you and Kelly ever talk about the menopause?' I ask, trying to veer things away from their theories about the likelihood of Vladimir Putin starting a nuclear war.

'What?' She splutters. 'Why would we talk about *that*?'

'Why not?'

'I'll tell you why not, Bryony. Because we don't waste our time focusing on silly little trends!'

'I don't think that the menopause is a trend, Mum.' I feel incredibly pompous, despite having been called out for using precisely this language myself just this morning. 'I think it's something that all women have been going through since the dawn of time.'

'Well, *exactly*, Bryony,' she says. 'Women have been going through the menopause since the dawn of time, so I really don't know why your generation has to bang on about it as if you discovered it. 'HRT this' and 'testosterone gel that'. Do you think

Margaret Thatcher would have been able to run the country if she'd complained every time she had a hot flush?'

'Maybe the country might have turned out a bit nicer if she had,' I snap.

'I mean, honestly, it's just part of life, isn't it? It's hardly worth talking about with my friends. We've got better things to be chatting about, social lives and the like.'

'How old were you when you went through the menopause?' I ask, undeterred.

'Bryony! What a question!'

'It's a perfectly reasonable one, Mum. It will help me be able to plan for my future. I mean, knowing what age you went through it means I can work out if there's time to give you more grandchildren.'

'If you must know, I didn't go through the menopause.'

'What? You mean you're still having periods at sev—'

'Bryony! That's quite enough, thank you very much! Now I need to go and walk the dog. Goodbye!'

Conversations with my mother: Part three

Three days later, she rings me back.

'About the menopause,' she says, very firmly. I imagine her closing her eyes to get through the embarrassment of having to talk about such *delicate* issues.

'Yes, Mum?'

'I had your brother at forty and then I never had a period again.' She speaks quickly, with purpose, like she just wants to get in and out of the conversation without anyone noticing she's there, an undercover spy disseminating crucial information about female reproductive health. 'Your grandmother went through it at forty-three. I've heard rumours that other female members of our family also experienced this process in their early forties. Now, let's never speak of this again.'

I feel like I am taking part in the forty-plus exam, which is like the eleven-plus, only for women approaching midlife.

Men don't have to take it, obviously. They can just cruise through to retirement without breaking a sweat. Certainly not a hot flush.

Here are some tester questions:

You go to the doctor to tell him about your perimenopause symptoms. Does he:
1. Respond in a kind and compassionate way, referring you for tests to gauge your levels of oestrogen and suggesting some helpful organisations and books that might be able to help as you start to navigate this journey?
2. Mansplain the menopause to you, pointing out that it is a natural process, not an illness, and that resources are obviously tight, so there's not a rat's chance in hell of being considered for HRT, but have you thought about mindfulness and meditation and losing some weight?

You tell the doctor that this seems to be his answer for everything. Does he:
1. Take your points on board, and have a long, thoughtful conversation with you about the woeful provision that exists in both women's health and mental health, suggesting that

185

he take these comments higher up to NHS management teams, so they can integrate the feedback into planning going forward?

2. Suggest antidepressants?

You explain that you are already on anti-depressants. Does he:

1. Apologise for not having looked properly at your records, explaining that government cuts mean he has to squeeze so much more work into his day?

2. Suggest you go private if you really believe you might be perimenopausal?

You go home feeling dejected, and a little confused about what is or isn't happening to you. Do you:

1. Call the doctor's surgery, ask for a second opinion, and then insist on being referred to a menopause specialist, as is your absolute right as a tax-paying citizen of the United Kingdom?

2. Obsess for hours over how weak you are for being in the midst of another breakdown, and for trying to use the menopause as an excuse for said weakness?

Your friend eventually encourages you to see a private menopause specialist. Do you:

1. Feel grateful that you are able to afford to do this, making a mental note to pass on some of this good fortune at a later date?

2. Berate yourself for being a stupid, white, privileged cis woman whose use of the private healthcare system is one of the reasons the country is in this mess in the first place?

The specialist Holly suggests I go and see is a real advert for the menopause. She has luminous, clear skin, bright eyes, a spring in her step. I look at her and think, *If that's what happens to me when my ovaries stop working, then bring it the fuck on.*

In contrast, I am sallow-skinned, with dark rings under my eyes. I feel broken. I feel incapable. Not in a self-pitying way, just in a factual one. By the time I wash up in her office in the spring of 2022, I am at a complete loss as to how I have managed to transport myself from my bed to her waiting room. The tiniest action – meeting someone other than Holly for a coffee, replying to a text or email – is beyond me. I have lost my mojo, although it seems a miracle that I ever had any in the first place. I know with absolute certainty that my husband hates me, my daughter has been damaged by me, and my boss is about to sack me. Everyone else . . . tolerates me. I wait for the summons from my editor, and analyse all the many ways in which I have failed the company during the pandemic by not being more productive, more enterprising, more enthusiastic. I google the names of my professional peers to see all the incredible things they have achieved, then use their amazing achievements as a stick with which to beat myself. I search for my name on a gossip forum known for its venom, and find a page of people saying things like, 'Bryony Gordon is insufferable' and 'Bryony Gordon really needs to write about something other than herself'. I pay attention to the nasty DMs that make their way into my inbox, and ignore the nice ones.

'Dear Ms Gordon, quite frankly, I find the contents of your writing repulsive, and I honestly believe it to be no exaggeration to say that it made me want to retch,' writes one person in response to a column about the benefits of exercise for mental health. 'The text was bad enough, but as for the photographs which accompanied the article ... words fail me. Let's just say that the whole sorry piece put me off my breakfast. Are you sure that you are in the right profession?'

I can't understand that these messages are rude, bordering on abusive, and that they say far more about the person who has sent them than they do about me. I just see evidence of all the truths that Jareth has spent years telling me. I am faulty, bad, a waste of space.

When I do get in touch with anyone, it is only because Jareth has started telling me they hate me, and I need to prove him wrong. My messages are needy, desperate, a little bit manipulative. If the person doesn't reply immediately, I become convinced that I have done something to upset them. I sit and scan my brain for all of the things I could have done wrong, all the misunderstandings that could have occurred to lead to this silence. Never mind that *I* frequently leave messages unanswered for weeks on end; I am, at this stage, beyond the point of rational thinking. My ego is in the penthouse, my self-esteem in the basement. I truly believe that I am a piece of shit the world revolves around.

The spin cycle of shame
(also known as: Washing Machine Brain)

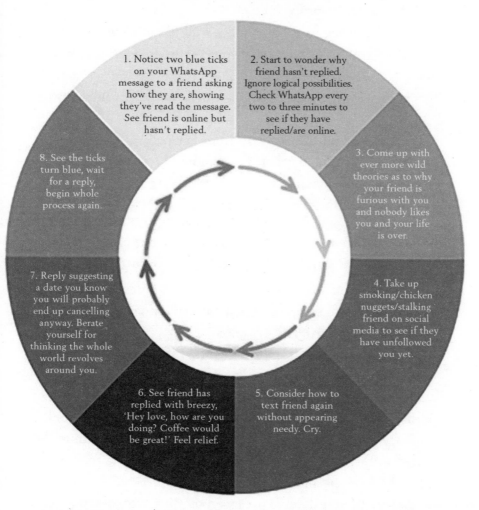

1. Notice two blue ticks on your WhatsApp message to a friend asking how they are, showing they've read the message. See friend is online but hasn't replied.

2. Start to wonder why friend hasn't replied. Ignore logical possibilities. Check WhatsApp every two to three minutes to see if they have replied/are online.

3. Come up with ever more wild theories as to why your friend is furious with you and nobody likes you and your life is over.

4. Take up smoking/chicken nuggets/stalking friend on social media to see if they have unfollowed you yet.

5. Consider how to text friend again without appearing needy. Cry.

6. See friend has replied with breezy, 'Hey love, how are you doing? Coffee would be great!' Feel relief.

7. Reply suggesting a date you know you will probably end up cancelling anyway. Berate yourself for thinking the whole world revolves around you.

8. See the ticks turn blue, wait for a reply, begin whole process again.

The menopause doctor asks me a series of questions about my health and lifestyle.

'Do you smoke?'

'Occasionally,' I lie.

'And what about alcohol – how often do you drink that?'

189

'Oh, never!' I beam, pleased to be getting an answer right. 'I'm sober.'

'What about your caffeine intake?'

My heart sinks. 'Well, you know, I do like my coffee.'

'How many cups a day would you say you drink?' She is making notes, not able to see the look of alarm that is spreading across my face as I try to work out how honest to be with her. 'One or two?'

'Um.'

'Three?' she says, looking up from her pad.

'I mean, I would say that it was more like four.'

'OK,' she says, taking notes.

'Sometimes five. Very, *very* rarely, six.'

I purse my lips and think about all the poor life decisions that have led me to turn my blood into espresso.

'Wow, that's quite a lot of coffee,' she says. 'You know, given your history of anxiety and obsessive compulsive disorder, I would say that cutting down on caffeine could be pretty life-changing for you. And as for smoking . . .'

'The thing is,' I start explaining, 'I've already had to give up quite a lot of fun things. You know, alcohol. Cocaine.'

She seems to have borrowed Peter's curious labrador face, or perhaps it is just one that gets handed out at medical school.

'Binge eating, that was the most recent one!' I continue. 'So coffee and cigarettes are kind of my thing. My little treat. I feel like I deserve *something*, right?'

'You think you deserve a cancerous stick that is almost certainly going to shorten your life?'

'Well, when you put it like that, it obviously doesn't sound quite so good.'

'The thing is, Bryony, a lot of people come to doctors hoping that they will give them a medicine that will solve all their

190

problems. HRT *can* be an amazing help, and it sounds as if you might benefit from it, especially given how young your mother was when she went through menopause.'

'I mean, my mum could be lying about how young she was,' I correct her. 'She doesn't like to speak about her age. When I turned twenty-seven, she told me *I* had to start lying about my age because she couldn't have a child older than—' I notice the bemused look on her face and realise I am rambling. I stop talking.

'Well, let's just assume she is telling you the truth. I think that a small amount of HRT would benefit you. We won't know, really, until we try. But I think a lot of other things are going to make a massive difference, too. Quitting smoking, at least cutting down on caffeine, if you can't quite cut it out. This is a time to think holistically about your health.'

'About the HRT.' I shift uncomfortably in my seat. 'I've heard it has risks of breast cancer attached. Could you talk to me about that?'

'OK, well, firstly, those studies took place decades ago, on much older women in their seventies. You're a woman in your early forties whose body should have oestrogen in it. There's no more in HRT than you would find in the contraceptive pill, and most women don't bat an eyelid at that. But also, if you're worried about getting cancer, then I would suggest that a more useful thing for you to do to assuage that anxiety would be to quit smoking.'

'Good point, well made.'

'We'll do a blood test so we can test your hormones, and then we'll take it from there, OK?'

I will do anything she tells me, if it stops me feeling like this. Except quit smoking and caffeine, of course.

'Fun' in your twenties and early thirties	'Fun' in your forties
Recreational drugs.	Ashwagandha and magnesium supplements.
Cigarettes.	Breathwork classes.
Booze.	A Symprove subscription.
Casual sex.	A wank.

They take the blood. They say it will be about three days before they get the results. I get in a taxi and cry all the way home about having to wait so long to find out what is wrong with me.

At home, I tell my husband he should leave me.

He doesn't *not* agree with me.

12

Dwayne 'The Rock' Johnson

It turns out my levels of oestrogen are pathetically low. There are caterpillars with more oestrogen than me. There are earwigs with more oestrogen than me. There are *men* with more oestrogen than me. Dwayne 'The Rock' Johnson has more oestrogen than me. This isn't what the doctor says, not exactly, but it is what I take from her reading of my blood-test results: in an oestrogen competition between me and Jason Statham, Statham would win – while doing pull-ups, obviously.

I am prescribed a low dose of HRT, to get started on. Every day, I am to spray a small amount of bio-identical oestrogen on to my arm. Fourteen days in, I will start taking progesterone tablets for the second half of my cycle, to help protect my womb.

'It can take up to three months before you really start to see a difference,' explains the doctor, and when I get off the Zoom, I start crying again.

Three months? At the moment, a minute feels like an hour, which feels like a day, which feels like a week, which feels like a month ... I don't know how I am going to get through the next three minutes, let alone the next three *months*.

I collect the HRT, walk home at pace, and tear open the packet containing the spray. I apply it. And then I wait.

About three days later, I wake up and I spring out of bed. I go downstairs, make myself a coffee, and start preparing breakfast for everyone. I turn on the radio, and switch it from Radio 4 to Heart, because I want to feel like the slightly naff forty-something I am. I dance around the kitchen to Taylor Swift's '. . . Ready For It?', because I am. I notice how easily my hips swing from side to side, and decide I would like to go and do some exercise.

'I'm going for a run!' I call upstairs after I've finished getting ready. 'I've left a pot of tea out and some cereal! See you later!'

It's raining, and I think how nice this is: that my first run back for months should be in the drizzle to keep me nice and cool. The first twenty minutes of my run are not hideous, which is strange, because the first twenty minutes of every run I've ever done are always hideous. I bounce along the common and it occurs to me how *natural* this feels. How non-gloopy. No wading through treacle today! I turn my face to the sky and smile as I feel the water land on my face.

'Thank you, universe,' I whisper into the air.

I get home and look at my diary for the day ahead, and I feel nothing other than a sense of vague interest that I have some Zoom meetings to do. *It would be so much nicer to do meetings face to face*, I think. *Now the restrictions have gone, I must make a mental note to suggest that I do all meetings in town from now on.* I chuckle to myself, because I am sure just the other day, the idea of even looking at my diary filled me with crushing fear.

Crushing fear? What's that?

I send an email to one of my editors and breezily suggest we meet up for lunch in the next couple of weeks. I WhatsApp

Holly and ask if she wants to go for a swim or hang out. While I'm there, I reply to a small portion of the dozens of messages that have sat unread in my inbox for the last few weeks. 'Sorry for late reply,' I type casually. 'I'm so rubbish at WhatsApp 😄'. I put a wash on, write 1,200 words, hang out the washing, then remember that I haven't done my post-run stretch. I sit on the floor in front of the big bay window in my bedroom, and as I put myself into pigeon pose, I realise two things:

1. The sun has come out.
2. I can do pigeon pose.

When did that happen?
I text Harry: 'Let's have sex tonight! ❤'
'???' he replies.
Aren't husbands funny?
I do some more writing, think about maybe making a big pasta bake for dinner, and google 'strength-training classes for women', because for some reason, today at least, strength-training feels like something I really want to try out. I mean, if I can do pigeon pose, who's to say I can't lift weights?
I call my mother and listen for a full twenty-seven minutes as she complains about Kelly, who has apparently started going for walks with someone called Sally who has a big house and a rich husband and an outdoor pool. And by the way, did I know that my father, from whom she has been divorced for two decades now, has decided not to come for Christmas?
It is April.
Oh, April, the most wonderful time of the year!
I pick up Edie from school, take her to the park, sit for an hour on a bench laughing with another mum about the general

197

cuteness of our children. Afterwards, we go for ice cream, just because.

'Are you OK?' asks Edie, when I tell her she can have two flavours instead of just the usual one.

'I'm fine my darling.' I smile, ruffling her head. 'I'm better than fine, actually. I'm glorious!'

And it's then that I realise I've gone through almost a whole day without Jareth piping up.

What the ...?

In all the time I've been writing about OCD and addiction, I've heard a lot of meteorology-based clichés concerning mental health. Some of them, I may even have said myself.

The sun will shine again.

The clouds will part.

You will weather this storm.

The sky may be dark now, but soon it will be blue again.

And so on and so forth.

But now, they are all true. Every single one of them. They're not just true – they are *gloriously* true. And I couldn't give a toss that they are clichés! Whereas just the other day, anything even remotely sentimental or mushy made me want to gag, now I think that sentimental and gushy is adorable. Cynicism, once a constant companion, appears to have fucked off. I am a walking, talking cliché and I couldn't be more delighted by it. After months and months of darkness, I feel a sudden lightness. My shoulders are no longer slumped. Yesterday, I was standing naked in a field, trying to fight off a hurricane. Today I am in the same field, but the sun is shining and I have a secure, strong house around me. It's not just that the weather has changed – so have my foundations. I actually *have* foundations, for a start. And clothes. I have those, too. I am basically a whole new person.

And there is only one thing that I've done differently.

HRT.

A week passes, and my energy stays buoyant. I notice my skin is brighter. I stop waking up drenched in sweat that has cooled on my skin. I go to sleep with ease. Jareth, Nigel and Jacob have moved out of my frontal lobe. I can hear vague chattering from them somewhere towards the back of my brain, but it's easy to tune out. I don't care enough to engage with them. The Stay Puft Marshmallow Man is long forgotten. I eat healthily without even giving it a second thought. My heart does no fluttering. For almost three weeks, I cannot believe it. I cannot believe that all this time, I have been suffering because I was low on a fucking hormone. All my problems have been solved, by a simple spray of oestrogen every morning.

Around eighteen days after I start taking HRT, I start crying.

And crying.

And crying.

And for the next few days, I barely stop.

It is almost impossible to describe what I am feeling in words, not least because to do so would require some sort of brain power, some sort of intelligence, some sort of basic ability, and I don't have any of that. It is as if a terrible sadness has filled my body. But not *just* a terrible sadness. There is also a terrible anger, and a terrible hopelessness, and a terrible sense of self-loathing. All the terribles, all vying terribly for space inside my terrible body.

As quickly as dark turned to light, it has switched back to

dark again. Only now, it's pitch fucking black. It's dark to the nth degree. It's the intergalactic void that exists between galaxies. It would be almost laughable if it weren't so fucking ... well, *dark*. And there is no space for self-awareness, anyway. It's all been crowded out by the need to sob, continuously, preferably while locked in a (dark) room on my own.

'You can't do that,' says Harry, when I try to explain to him why I can't get out of bed of a morning. 'You can't lock yourself away in a room by yourself, because that would be giving in.'

'This isn't a fucking Hollywood movie,' I somehow manage to snivel from under the bed. 'I'm not some Avenger whose defeat at the hands of Thanos is going to result in the world ending.'

'Bryony,' he says, sitting down on the bed next to me. 'We've been here before.'

'What do you mean by that?'

'You know what I mean. I mean, you know that this is the OCD and the depression speaking. And that you have to fight back, or it will just get worse.'

'I'm sorry that I'm so fucking tiresome with my endless issues that interrupt your day.'

'Don't be like that.'

'Please just make sure Edie gets to school without seeing me like this, and then leave me alone.'

I know as I am saying it that I am being completely unreasonable. I know that I am being self-pitying. I know that I am being selfish. I know that I am failing to carry out even the most basic of my responsibilities. I know that I should get up, and do all the things I have agreed to do. I know that if I get out of bed and leave the house, I will feel better. I know that a decent human being would get up out of their pity pit, but I also know that I am not a decent human being. I know that I am a bad mother and a crummy wife and a shit employee, and that things would be better for everyone if I simply ceased to exist.

But I also know this: if I had a physical condition that flared up periodically, leaving me bed bound, my husband would not have just walked out of the room rolling his eyes, wishing I would pull myself together.

Things you know about depression that make absolutely fuck-all difference when you have depression

- Depression makes it hard to get out of bed because if you're in bed, the illness has it where it wants you: alone.
- Depression thrives in isolation, because then it's less likely to be made better by the balm of connection.
- Depression tells you that you don't have depression, and you're just a dickhead.
- Depression can make you feel listless, paranoid and hopeless.
- Depression can lead to forgetfulness, mostly about the symptoms of depression

To be fair to Harry, even I am tired of myself by this point. By my calculations, things have been not quite right for almost two years now, if you include the binge eating and the rampant, almost deranged denial that anything was wrong, which most psychological professionals definitely would. And two years is quite a long time to be in denial, especially when you are someone who is supposed to have a vague awareness of how mental health works. It is, to be precise, twenty-four months of wallowing around in self-pity; 730 days of thinking about very little other than my own uselessness; 17,520 hours of wondering what's wrong with me; 1,051,200 minutes thinking about all the ways in which people might hate me. If only I could tell them: 'Believe me, none of you hate me as much as I do myself!'

In a cruel twist of fate, my iPhone chooses the arrival of this intergalactic void to remind me of our trip to Thailand at the end of 2019/beginning of 2020. 'For you: Phuket, 2019 trip' flashes up on my screen as I try to fight the terribles that day. I decide to watch, knowing that to do so will be like picking at a scab. Good. I'm in the mood for some blood and gore.

Images of me looking happy on a beach begin flashing up on my screen to a background of twee music. Who the fuck does my iPhone think it is? Davina McCall showing me my best bits after I've been booted off *Big Brother*? It's one minute and forty-six seconds of saccharine snapshots from my life Before Covid, when I had everything except the self-awareness to realise that every last bit of luck I had was just that: luck. A fluke. Throw the dice again and watch as all that contentment you fought so hard for gets pulled out from under you like a rug.

'Stop being so self-pitying,' says Jareth.

'Yes, you're being a bit self-indulgent,' agrees Nigel.

'That's the problem with you, Bryony,' lectures Jacob. 'It's all about *you*.'

The Stay Puft Marshmallow Man doesn't say anything. He just hands me a packet of cooking chorizo.

I try to convince myself that this heaviness is a blip. A small glitch, the kind that the doctor warned me about. The HRT could take up to three months to work, she'd told me, and I had felt amazing within three days. Perhaps a couple of wobbly moments here and there are to be expected? I just need to buckle up and ride this out. Woman up, if you will.

I go to see the personal trainer I booked during my brief moment of sunshine a few weeks ago. Perhaps, if HRT isn't the magic cure to all my ills, then strength-training will be? I've heard that as a perimenopausal woman, it is extremely important to do weights, because on top of menopause taking away all your joy and hard-won self-esteem, it also takes away your bone density. Which leads me to wonder: if the menopause taketh with one hand (and, oh boy, does it taketh), what, exactly does it giveth with the other?

The personal trainer is based at a gym only a short walk away from my house, because I have learned by this point that if I try to do anything beyond my postcode, I become so overwhelmed with fear that I will almost always end up chickening out and cancelling the thing. But as I walk the ten minutes to the gym, I realise that actually, I need to readjust the allowable distance for social events: from my postcode, to my house.

With each step away from my home, I experience the very real fear that if I carry on, I will never be able to turn back. I will never be able to turn back because the house will burn down, or the taps will have been left running and the ceiling will fall through, or because the police will show up with evidence of how awful I am and Harry will not want to ever let me back in.

BG News is back on, and the volume has been turned up to max.

Nigel Farage: On today's episode, can you ever properly atone for your sins with sobriety?

Jacob Rees-Mogg: While many claim that everyone deserves a second chance, is some behaviour unforgivable? We'll hear more from our brave whistle-blower, Jareth the Goblin King, who has experienced first-hand why it's a bad idea to trust a self-confessed alcoholic with no shame.

'FUCK OFF, JARETH!' I scream out loud, as I pass the bus stop. Luckily I have my AirPods in, so it looks as if I am simply having a heated argument with an elaborately named boyfriend. A woman looks at me with sympathy, and perhaps the merest suggestion in her eyes that I dump this loser with a strange name. 'I've been trying for three decades,' I want to cry. 'I've been trying!'

By the time I arrive at the gym, I am already exhausted, and I haven't lifted anything other than the weight of the world – which exists entirely in my own head. Perhaps this cavalcade of mental health issues will make excellent training for what I am about to do, and result in an unlikely new career as an Olympic weightlifter?

'Why are you so fucking ridiculous?' sneers Jareth.

The personal trainer is friendly and welcoming, but I can feel the walls coming in on me. The tinny dance music played over the speakers seems to have been created at exactly the right pitch to fuck with my brain. The warm-ups appear to have been concocted with the sole purpose of annoying me. The other people in the gym seem to have been placed there only to make me feel fat. I grit my teeth and do what I am told, but I can feel the Lycra digging into my stomach, the underwiring of my sports bra digging into my ribs, the judgement of Jareth closing around my windpipe.

Quite out of nowhere, I wish I could self-combust with rage.

I take a deep breath, scared by my anger.

'Now we are going to try some skull-crushers,' says my trainer, brightly.

'Some *what?*' I splutter.

'Skull-crushers. Don't worry, they're not as frightening as they sound!'

Everything is exactly as frightening as it sounds.

He talks me through what I will be doing: a 'simple' tricep extension with some light weights, while lying on the floor.

I offer a feeble joke in the hope it will lighten my mood. 'Lying on the floor, I *can* do.' I get on to the mat, and he hands me a pair of dumbbells that weigh no more than a couple of kilos each. I start bending and extending my elbows as instructed, and as I do this, I realise I can block out the dance music with pure fucking exertion. I can almost ignore the taunts from Jareth that I am fat and ugly and probably a serial-killing paedophile to boot. I ask for heavier weights, with the notion that these might stop the noise entirely, that I might actually be able to use them to cave Jareth's head in. The trainer leaps up enthusiastically and gets some new dumbbells, and I imagine clubbing Jareth over the head with them. I bend and extend, bend and extend, and it is only when I finish the set that I realise I am sobbing.

'Are you OK?' I hear the trainer asking from above me.

I put the weights to one side and sit up.

'No,' I say, getting to my feet. 'No, I don't think I am. I'm sorry, I think I need to leave.'

I make my excuses and run home to the safety of the empty house. No fire. No floods. No police. Just the chaos of my own head.

How to get strong!

A guide to strength-training for beginners

- Remember, you have as much right to be in a gym as anyone else.
- Gym equipment and weights do not exclusively belong to men with bulging biceps, six-packs and every item from the latest Gymshark collection.

- Men with bulging biceps, six-packs and every item from the latest Gymshark collection don't always make the best personal trainers.
- When looking for a strength-trainer, remember that *you* are allowed to choose – you don't have to go with the first oiled-up gym bro who walks into your line of vision when you sign up at Fitness First.
- The best PT I've ever had was a woman.
- So was the second best.
- You don't have to exercise to be the strongest or the fastest or the fittest. You can exercise to be the happiest.
- Exercise isn't about the losses – the inches around your waist, the number on the scales – but the gains: the clarity, the time to yourself, the endorphins, the community in which you find yourself.
- Nobody ever *wants* to go to the gym, but nobody ever regrets going to the gym.

The menopause specialist says that it sounds as if I am intolerant to progesterone.

'Oh,' I say, not quite understanding.

'Progesterone intolerance is when you are sensitive to progesterone,' explains the doctor. 'Or more likely, its synthetic version. The majority of women actually find progesterone relaxing and calming.' She smiles, as if she is telling me an interesting titbit that I might like to pass on to friends, or retell at a dinner party. 'That's why we tell you to take it at night. But about one in ten women find it has the opposite effect. It can cause panic attacks, anxiety, irritability, that kind of thing.'

I stay silent, the alternative being me shouting: 'AND YOU THOUGHT NOT TO TELL ME THIS *WHY*, EXACTLY?'

'It can also cause forgetfulness and heightened emotions. The physical symptoms of it tend to be acne, greasy skin, bloating, dizziness, breast tenderness . . .'

'Wow, menopause really is the gift that keeps on taking.'

'But don't worry!' she trills. 'It's usually very easy to deal with. Instead of taking the progesterone orally, you can insert it into your vagina.'

'Right,' I say, trying to seem completely unfazed by this suggestion.

'It's off-licence to take it this way, but then most things are when it comes to treating the menopause.'

'Off-licence?' I say, confused. I haven't heard that term for a while.

'It means that the National Institute for Health and Care Excellence haven't OKed it for use on the NHS, even though it's perfectly safe. It's just a consequence of nobody really caring that much about menopause treatment.' She shrugs her shoulders nonchalantly. 'They've sort of "forgotten" to give any of the treatment proper authorisation.'

'Seems entirely reasonable.' I wince.

'Nothing to be worried about, though. Most women in America insert progesterone vaginally. We think it's better that way, as it means the hormone acts locally, where it's supposed to actually have an effect, as opposed to going through your whole system. Taking it orally, as is licensed, means that women such as yourself can feel the effects more in their brains.'

'It's like I've woken up and realised that all women over the age of fifty deserve damehoods,' I say, trying to make light of this.

'Oh, believe me, one day, we're going to look back on the way we deal with menopause now and be absolutely appalled.' She shakes her head. 'We are very dismissive of hormones, or at

207

least the ones that effect women. But hormones are the most powerful chemicals known to human kind, and shouldn't be underestimated. Especially when it comes to something like mental health.'

On my way home, I call Holly in disbelief.

'Did you know that most of the treatment for the menopause has to be done off-licence because at no point has our medical establishment thought it a good idea to make perfectly safe medicine available to women going through the menopause?'

'Newsflash, Bryony,' she says sarcastically, as if I have just called to tell her that the sun rises in the east and sets in the west. 'There's a lot you're about to learn about women's health, sweetie-pie. For example, if you try and get your health insurance company to cover any of your appointments with a private menopause doctor, they will probably laugh at you. Or tell you to fuck off.'

'You're not serious?'

'Well, no, they probably won't tell you to fuck off. But it's not far off that.' I can almost see the arch look on Holly's face down the phone. 'We're lucky to have HRT at all, you know, what with all the shortages. I had to go to seven different pharmacies the other day to get my HRT gel. You'd think I was trying to find one of Willy Wonka's golden tickets – except instead of a lifetime's supply of chocolate, I get the chance to feel vaguely normal for three days rather than wanting to murder my colleagues.'

'I reckon that if men had ovaries, there's no way this shit would happen.' I light a cigarette, and puff in rage. 'Like, there's absolutely no way that they'd put up with HRT shortages. Everything from tampons to sanitary towels to the gel would be free. You know how people complain that we wang on about the menopause too much now? If men went through it, you can

208

bet your bottom dollar that we'd all have to talk about it for at least eighty per cent of each day, with the remaining twenty per cent given over to pampering men going through it. There'd be a Minister for Periods and a Minister for Menopause. They'd dedicate entire sessions of Prime Minister's Questions to it. There'd be a weekly magazine show presented by Jeremy Clarkson that would involve road-testing all the latest in menstrual technology. Netflix would have entire categories dedicated to menopause. Boots would not call the tampon aisle "feminine hygiene" and hide it at the back. They would call it "MASCULINE MARVEL-LOUSNESS" and have tampons decorating the shop windows like fairy lights. And men going to get HRT would *not* end up feeling as if they're trying to procure crystal meth from the dark web. I mean, I've done drug deals that felt less dodgy than that appointment just now.'

'Tell me about it, Bryony, tell me about it.'

I take her literally. 'Like, there was one time that I had been waiting at a work Christmas party for two hours for a coke dealer to turn up, and when he finally texted to say that he had arrived, the bloody books editor stopped me in the stairwell to have a nice long chat about where I was planning to spend Christmas. I could have murdered him! Then, when I eventually got out of the venue and on to the street, I was greeted by the sight of the police swooping on said dealer's car. I ended up being pretty grateful for that books editor, let me tell you.'

It's time to play . . .
Drug Dealer or Menopause Doctor?

- 'I've got this new product from Australia that's supposed to be amazing for lifting your mood and energy.' (Answer: Menopause doctor)
- 'Try this, and if you like it, we can get you more.' (Answer: Menopause doctor)
- 'You're not supposed to take it this way, but trust me, it works better and won't do you any harm.' (Answer: Menopause doctor)
- 'You should rub it on your clitoris for the best effects.' (Answer: Menopause doctor)

'What are you on about, Bryony?'

'I'm not sure. I can't even remember what we were talking about.'

'I think it was menopause,' prompts Holly, though she sounds unsure herself.

'Oh yes! Menopause! Even the dodgiest of drug deals have felt less seedy than the doctor telling me just then that I should shove the progesterone pills up my fanny, but not to go around shouting about it. As if I'm going to go live on Instagram of an evening as I'm inserting them into my hoo-ha.'

'So that's her solution to the crashing depression and thoughts of suicide?'

'Yep.' I inhale deeply. 'Shove a pill up my vagina, and think of England.'

'It could be worse,' says Holly.

'I'm not sure how.'

13

I think I might be dying
(for real)

Snapshot from my iPhone's Notes app, May 2022

20:54　　　　　　　　　　　.ıl 📶 38

❮ Notes　　　　　　　　　　　　　　　⬆️ ⋯

Things to buy:

- a kettlebell
- one of those mats with nails in them that you lie on
- crystals???
- concealer

      ☑️　　📷　　Ⓐ　　✏️

A few weeks later, I find out. The progesterone has exactly the same effect on me when I insert it vaginally as it did orally. Within days of pushing the not-so-little pill into my vagina, I learn two things:

- That much of it falls out into the toilet the next day.
- What doesn't fall out leaves me feeling suicidal.

The doctor says we can try a different type of progesterone. Then, when that doesn't make any difference, she says that I can try having more oestrogen, which she thinks might offset the effects of the progesterone. Months pass; things get worse. I begin to think I am losing my mind. Eventually, I break down during a Zoom call with her. I cannot take progesterone for a moment more. Whatever life is like without it, it can't be worse than this.

The doctor starts talking about something called PMDD, which leaves me with a blank face.

'It stands for premenstrual dysphoric disorder,' she explains. 'It's like PMS, only more serious. It causes really severe anxiety and depression in the two weeks before your period starts, we think because of an intolerance to progesterone. I'm wondering if maybe it's something you might have experienced before.'

'I don't know,' I say truthfully. 'It's only really since I got sober that I've properly started paying attention to my menstrual cycle, to my body. I got my period when I was twelve, I guess, and then I started drinking at about fourteen, and to be honest, I was more or less permanently out of it, aside from when I was pregnant, until the age of thirty-seven. I've always thought of PMS as cramping and a bit of snappiness, but I've never really had cramping, and the snappiness was something I always put down to being tired and hungover. So I never saw my periods as a problem. I always just thought *I* was the problem, you know?'

The doctor is respectful enough to not say anything for a time. To let those words sink in for me. Then she asks, 'How old were you when you first started experiencing OCD badly, would you say?'

214

I think about the alien pregnancy, and the fear I had AIDS. 'I was twelve,' I whisper.

'And you got your period at?'

'Twelve.' I breathe out. I think about how the OCD came out of nowhere and disappeared just as quickly a few months later. Was my body just more used to the hormones?

'And how was your mental health during pregnancy?' she asks, politely.

'Absolutely fucking shocking, if you will pardon my language.'

'Well, that would tally, given that your body is absolutely flooded with progesterone during pregnancy.' She looks up at me, and begins to talk softly. 'Listen, the chances are that you have always been the kind of person more prone to mental health issues. The hormones aren't the *cause* of your OCD. But they could certainly be exacerbating it. It would make sense, given that the condition first flared up badly around the same time your periods started, and that it suddenly flared up again earlier this year. Both are times when your hormones are fluctuating and out of sync, which could explain why the episode you have just had was so severe and seemed so out of the blue. As I've said to you before, hormones have a huge impact on mental health.'

'So what can I do about it?' I ask, feeling slightly forlorn.

'Well, you have to have progesterone. It protects your womb. I want to suggest we try you on the Intrauterine system (IUS). It gets inserted into your womb, where it secretes a small amount of progesterone locally. It can be used as birth control, but it is also used in HRT, especially with women like you who have trouble tolerating progesterone.'

'But I don't understand,' I say. 'How is having progesterone permanently in my body going to make me feel better? Surely it's going to be worse?'

215

'We think that because it's directly in your womb, it has even less effect than it does in your vagina. You may get symptoms for around three months, but they tend to go after that. Your body gets used to it. There are women I know who are progesterone intolerant, and whose lives have been transformed by the IUS.'

'And what are the options if the IUS doesn't work?'

'Well, you have to have progesterone if you have a womb,' she says. 'So if you can't deal with progesterone at all, then you will have to have a hysterectomy.'

'Seems entirely reasonable,' I quip, but I'm the only one who is laughing, and I'm not quite sure why.

Conditions women have suffered from since the beginning of time that we are only talking about now

Endometriosis: A serious condition whereby tissue similar to the lining of the uterus grows outside the uterus. Can cause severe pain and make it harder to get pregnant.

Fibroids: Growths in your uterus that are almost always benign, but can cause heavy bleeding, pelvic pain and bloating.

Adenomyosis: When displaced tissue grows into the wall of the uterus. Can lead to difficulty conceiving and mis-carriage.

Dysmenorrhea: Extremely painful periods.

Menorrhagia: Extremely heavy bleeding during your periods.

Polycystic ovary syndrome (PCOS): A condition that affects how the ovaries work, which can cause irregular periods, excess body hair, weight gain, and in some cases infertility.

> **Stress incontinence:** Weeing without meaning to. Sometimes caused by childbirth.

I go away and cry. I feel like a freak, or a guinea pig. A freaky guinea pig? There is a lot to unpack here. Firstly, that my hormones have probably been making my life difficult for as long as I can remember; secondly, that because of my sex, this was never seen as something important enough to investigate; thirdly, that if I want to feel better, things are probably going to have to get much worse first as my body adjusts to the IUS; fourthly, that if my body *doesn't* adjust to the IUS, I will have to have a pretty large part of it ripped out in an operation that will have other, different consequences for me; fifthly (is that even a word? My menopausal brain seems to have lost the ability to string sentences together), this entire process will at best take up the next few months of my life, at worst the next year.

I realise I am lucky, because I have my darling daughter and because, despite what I tell my mother every time she asks when we are going to have another, Harry and I long ago agreed that we only wanted one child. This hasn't ruined any hopes or dreams that I may have been harbouring for a bigger family. I have a supportive husband, and a workplace that is understanding because of the nature of what I write about. I have money, resources, and a network of people around me, including Peter and my twelve-step meetings, and Naomi if I need her. I have this private menopause doctor whom I can afford to see, and who will give me the very best care available, even if that care might have to come off-licence. I am, by all accounts, exceedingly fortunate, even if I have spent the best part of the last year wanting to kill myself.

But I think of all the many women going through a difficult menopause who aren't so lucky. Those who might have wanted

217

kids but not have managed it because of the incredible pressures society puts on women to 'have it all'; those who might have been fobbed off by their GPs and shoved on antidepressants; those who might be crippled by symptoms but expected to get on with it with no support from employers. This, I realise, is the landscape in which women are still expected to live in late 2022: one where those able to access care for debilitating conditions – conditions that, under any other circumstances, would not be tolerated – are made to feel 'lucky'.

And perhaps because of this, there is a voice in the back of my head that wants to berate me for being so weak. Surely if the menopause caused such awful, awful side effects, we would take it more seriously? So perhaps this isn't the menopause. Perhaps I'm just jumping on a bandwagon. Perhaps, as ever, the real problem is me.

I look up premenstrual dysphoric disorder (PMDD). The Johns Hopkins Medicine School, one of the most prestigious health-care centres in America, describes it as: 'A much more severe form of premenstrual syndrome (PMS). It may affect women of childbearing age. It's a severe and chronic medical condition that needs attention and treatment. Lifestyle changes and sometimes medicines can help manage symptoms.'

These symptoms usually appear during the week before men-struation, and end within a few days of your period starting. They are bad enough, the Johns Hopkins website notes, to 'disrupt daily living tasks. Symptoms of PMDD are so severe that women have trouble functioning at home, at work, and in relationships during this time. This is markedly different than other times during the month.'

The symptoms are many and varied, and the majority of them

are psychological. Once more, they read like a laundry list of everything that has been happening in my life for the last few months, and certainly at other times in my life when I have been close to the edge: irritability; nervousness; lack of control; agitation; anger; insomnia; difficulty concentrating; depression; severe fatigue; anxiety; confusion; forgetfulness; poor self-image; paranoia; emotional sensitivity; crying spells; moodiness; trouble sleeping; appetite changes; food cravings; diminished sex drive. Then there is a host of physical symptoms so wide-ranging that you would never think to link them to your hormones and periods: allergies; respiratory infections; vomiting; skin inflammation with itching; aggravation of other skin disorders, including cold sores; diminished urination; vision changes; eye infections; decreased coordination; headaches; dizziness; fainting; numbness, prickling, tingling or heightened sensitivity of arms and/or legs; muscle spasms; easy bruising; *heart palpitations*.

I am hesitant to be a Google doctor and diagnose myself with PMDD, and I am loath to be the kind of person who blames all their many psychological problems on one single thing. But given that there are barely any diagnostic tests available for the condition (nobody has bothered to develop them), I'm going to have to take a stab in the dark and diagnose myself. And as I read more about PMDD, it is hard to ignore the fact that it might have had *something* to do with my troubles over the years.

I think about a parallel universe, one where women's health is taken seriously, and wonder how different things might have been for me. Might my mother have put two and two together when she saw my mental health spiralling at around the same time I got my first period? Might my father have also noticed, this being a parallel universe where we *all* take female health seriously? Might I have gone to the doctor, who would have been able to counsel me on ways to manage my health? Might there have been proper research into PMDD, and female hormones generally, that would mean there was a wealth of treatments available to people who found themselves at the sharp end of this? With proper healthcare systems in place, not to mention better education about emotional wellbeing, might I have avoided alcoholism and addiction and found healthier ways to cope? With more time to pursue hobbies and interests, might women have been more able to get on with things like, I dunno, ruling the fucking world?

Instead, we live in a universe where the only treatment for PMDD is to get the fuck on with it and stop whingeing, that gaslighting voice of the patriarchy being so all-encompassing that often, we genuinely believe it to be our own.

I know I am going to have to get the IUS inserted, but I am terrified. The thought of a constant drip-drip of progesterone inside me sends me into a panic. At the moment, I have a week or so of respite, during the bit of the HRT cycle when you only take oestrogen, and those days are like manna from heaven for me. But the two weeks taking progesterone are genuine hell. This is not an exaggeration. I am constantly teary, always paranoid. I believe with every fibre of my being that my career is over, squandered because of my many, many failings. I look for meaning where there is none, in a slightly short exchange with a colleague, or an email from an editor that does not include a kiss. Didn't they used to put kisses on everything, before my career was over? I search through old emails to check, and get sucked into reading old conversation chains where I realise with horror that I was flaky and non-committal and filed my copy late. I wonder how I ever managed to get away with it, 'it' being the endless shortcomings that somehow make up my character.

I start to make plans for when I lose my job, or have to resign because I am incapable of handling the stress anymore. I think about how long my savings will last me – two weeks, tops – and start to look on Rightmove for parts of the UK where we could afford to live mortgage-free if we sold our matchbox home in south London. I make calculations, forecasts for worst-case scenarios. I think of all the frankly *indulgent* things on which I have frittered away money: drugs, alcohol, clothes, holidays, make-up, take-aways, cooking chorizo, Netflix, overdrafts, sheet masks, dry robes. I imagine all the tubes of toothpaste and moisturiser that I could have made last longer if I had squeezed them properly and cut them in half to scoop out every last bit. I think of all the messages I haven't replied to, and all the people who are disappointed in me.

I am like the girl in the *Black Mirror* episode whose approval rating keeps slipping ever lower, only not quite as beautiful. I start to see myself not as a human, but as an object bereft of value. I feel like a once-glittering brooch that has lost all of its worth, relegated to a dusty box in the back of a cupboard where it will be forgotten about. I wonder if everything would be made better by Botox, or fillers? Maybe things would be better if I was thinner? Maybe things would be better if more men wanted to have sex with me? If any man at all wanted to?

There are moments when I consider the other options, the ones that are not meant to be considered. It's not so much that I want to die, more that it feels too exhausting to keep living. Sometimes I feel nothing, and those times, I suppose, are the good bits. When I feel nothing, I try to get on with work. It rarely lasts long. There I will be, sitting at my desk, trying to answer emails, when all of a sudden I will be overwhelmed with the realisation that life is pointless and I am futile, and everything I am doing is utterly meaningless.

So that's fun.

Peter says I am deluded. He says that my view of reality does not match anyone else's. He says that instead of experiencing delusions of grandeur, I am experiencing delusions of inferiority.

'In twelve-step programmes, we talk a lot about ego, right?' he says.

I nod.

'And in conventional terms, out there in the real world, we think of someone with a big ego as being really in love with themselves right?'

I nod.

'When actually, everyone has an ego. It's the part we develop to bridge the gap between the conscious and the sub-conscious. Someone can be caught up in their ego and really hate themselves. Ego is just the bit of us concerned with the self. It can make us think we have a bigger effect on people than we actually do, be that positive or negative. It assumes that everyone else isn't busy in their own ego – which, unless they're a Buddhist monk, they probably are. By the sounds of it, you spend most of your time at the moment thinking about how awful you are, how miserable you make everyone.

'But Bryony, no one human can have that effect on anyone else, unless perhaps they're Vladimir Putin, and you're absolutely not that. Nobody is thinking about how awful you are, nobody is thinking that you're over, and if they are, they've got problems of their own. You're in a sort of twilight zone right now, where you're not thinking straight. You're unwell.'

'I'm unwell.' I nod.

It sounds better than saying I'm fine.

As Christmas approaches, I decide to bite the bullet and book in for the coil. It can't be any worse than this, surely? Just to be certain, I google things like 'IUS OCD menopause' and 'IUS anxiety'. The sites I find do not reassure me that the path I am on leads to sunny uplands.

Online, I find many other women who have, like me, had breakdowns while also experiencing the menopause. Hundreds if not thousands of them, all reduced to passing information between each other on internet forums where nobody will shush them for wanging on too much about the menopause.

Menoforums

@periperimenochick: I had the IUS put in, and within days I was so angry I could barely function. When I tried to get an appointment with my doctor to have it taken out, I was told I would have to wait three weeks, and I'm sorry but that was NOT happening, so I am even more sorry to say that I downed three strong gin and tonics, ran a bath, and pulled it out myself.

@fedup: The IUS is evil. It turned me into a different person. My husband almost divorced me. I don't understand how it is allowed???? Like, in what universe is it acceptable to let women go through this? Big Pharma should be ashamed. Or at least be forced to pay the fees for my divorce lawyer, lol.

@constantpainjane: I had the IUS because the doctor said it would make my periods lighter, and maybe even stop them. That sounded good to me, because the reason I worked out I was in perimenopause was that instead of my periods disappearing or becoming less frequent, I had the opposite happen. My periods became much, much heavier and much, much longer, and it was just horrible. So I had high hopes for the IUS – no more periods??? BRING IT ON! Well, I am sorry, but from the moment I had it put in – bloody painful – I did not stop bleeding. I was told it would probably settle down or stop after three to six months, but it just went on and on, and I had to get it taken out. If you want my advice, don't touch it with a bargepole.

@menomaiden1976: You know how they say it's a simple procedure and you'll be able to go back to work straight afterwards? Maybe if your job is testing mattresses. Honestly, the 'procedure' was more like an operation. They should totally offer you general anaesthetic. I screamed so loudly that the nurse had to go and apologise to the people in the waiting room. I practically had to get an ambulance home (well, an Uber), and then I couldn't do anything for, like, a week after? Worked a treat for me otherwise, though.

@felicityflowers52: My husband said he could feel the strings, which was when I realised how the IUS worked as a contraceptive.

The private menopause doctor has told me that I should be able to get the coil for free through my GP, but when I call to enquire about this, the man on reception seems confused.

'Sorry, you want what?'

'The IUS. It's a form of contraception,' I say.

'Hmm, not heard of it,' says the bloke on the other end of the

224

line. 'Hang on one sec.' I hear him put his hand over the phone receiver in an attempt to mute his conversation. It doesn't work. 'Janet? JANET? There's a lady here who says she wants us to put in a coil or something? Some type of contraception? You what? Yeah, I thought so.' He removes his hand from the receiver. 'We don't do contraception here. You have to call the people who do the tests for STIs – what's that, Janet? The South London Sexual Health services, apparently. I can google the number for you, or you can do it yourself.'

'I'll do it myself, thanks.'

I google the number, call it, and am put on hold for an interminable amount of time that could be twenty-seven minutes, or twenty-seven days. When I finally get through, the woman tells me that the next available appointment is in March. I thank her for her time and wonder if a man faced with an equivalent situation would be this patient, or polite.

Another internet search: this time, to find out how much it costs to have an IUS fitted privately. A company in Harley Street quotes me £500 for the coil fitting, but explains that I will also need to book in for a £1,000 new patient consultation. Eventually, I find somewhere that will do it for £275, which feels like a bargain, like getting a Chanel handbag on the cheap, only far less pleasurable.

Edith from the practice calls me and talks me through the procedure. 'Take some paracetamol, take the rest of the day off, and remember that you can't have a bath or do any heavy exercise for one week after the coil has been fitted.'

'I don't do heavy exercise,' I say, 'so that won't be a problem.'

'Yes, it is rarely something our patients complain about!' Edith seems delighted at the opportunity to make a joke, and for the first time in what feels like months and months, her delight sparks something in me. 'And as for when I tell women they won't be able to have sex for a week or so – well, it depends on their marital status how happy they are about that.'

'Ha!' I laugh, and realise it is the first time I have done this involuntarily for eons. 'Edith, can I ask you something?'

'Ask me anything you want, my love. Unless it's about politics. I'm about to eat my lunch and don't want my stomach turned.'

'I promise you it's not about politics.' I smile. 'I just wondered, is having the coil put in really horrible?'

'Darling, many things are horrible in this life. You only have to turn on the news to see that. Having an IUS put in is fine, in the grand scheme of things. A little bit of pain for a whole lot of gain.'

'I'm intolerant to progesterone, so I'm a bit scared of it,' I find myself explaining. 'I'm worried it will make me go loopy. Or even *more* loopy, perhaps I should say.'

'My dear, sometimes I think the loopy among us are actually the most sane. Look at this world. Who wouldn't lose their minds? But in all seriousness, I know this time of life can be troublesome. I've been there myself, I'll have you know. But as someone far wiser than me once said, it is always darkest before the dawn.'

'There's a song that says that, by Florence and the Machine.' I feel a shiver go up my spine. 'I heard it one day, when I was trying to get sober. It was like she was singing to me, telling me it was going to be OK.'

'And was it OK? Did you get sober?'

'I did.' I nod. 'I did. I got five years in the summer.'

'Wonderful! So there you have it. You got sober. You can easily see off a measly little thing like the IUS.'

'I hope you're right, Edith,' I say. 'I hope you're right.'

14

Welcome to my womb

Snapshot from my iPhone's Notes app, December 2022

23:27

< Notes

Hard things I have survived that will surely make getting the coil a piece of piss in comparison
- rehab
- umpteen OCD breakdowns
- two marathons, one in only my underwear
- that triathlon where I came second to last
- interviewing Joan Collins while I was on a comedown

The appointment is scheduled for mid to late January, which is not ideal, but also not March. Somehow, I get through Christmas without doing anything stupid. I smile. I laugh. I eat a lot of roast potatoes dipped in bread sauce. I make sure my daughter has lots of presents. I see in the new year with friends in Cornwall, where I fantasise about what it would be like to just ... live here, off the land? But I have a job, responsibilities. A mortgage that's visible from space. Also, in the first week of the new year, I am due to go to California to interview Prince Harry about his new book, which feels like a strange detour into a life I used to live. It is like I am dreaming. I keep expecting the trip to be cancelled, for his team to call me up and tell me that there's been a terrible mistake, that he thought he was being interviewed by the Bryony he first met in 2016, the vibrant, interesting one, not the menopausal, weeping version that exists in early 2023.

I sign an NDA that prohibits me from revealing anything about the book ahead of its publication. I am sent a password-protected PDF of the book that frightens me. I want to call up the publishers and tell them to cancel the interview; I am not good enough to do it and I will only fuck it up. It would be much better if they gave it to one of the many better journalists out there who are doing more interesting work than I am.

Things you still have to do while trying to set up an interview with Prince Harry:

- Take your child to the doctor to get antibiotics.
- Clean out the guinea pig's cage.
- Find your passport.
- Kegels.

My daughter has an ear infection. I want only to crawl into bed with her and stroke her head and rub her feet and make her feel better. I think: if I could create a world where me, my husband and Edie could live by the sea without the need for any of *this*, then that would be heaven to me.

Instead, I kiss her goodbye, promise to get her a big present, and make my way to the airport, thinking about all the ways in which the plane might end up crashing into the sea. I spend the entire eleven-hour flight to Los Angeles worrying that I am a bad mother. In LA, it is raining in a way that it never rains in LA. Prince Harry's press person calls me to say there are landslide warnings near his home in Montecito, and that we might have to do the interview somewhere else. I try to sleep, but the newspaper I work for keeps calling me in the middle of the night, asking if there is anything in the book I can tell them about. I mention the NDA, and wonder why I do what I do when really I just want to live by the sea with my family. Then I lie awake, worrying I am a bad journalist who deserves to be sacked.

We end up going to Montecito, where I sit by a fire with Prince Harry and find myself fighting my brain, which either wants to fall asleep, or forget what it was talking about just a minute ago. I try to grab at words that are on the tip of my tongue; I think of profound, pertinent questions that I lose a moment later, banished forever by my menopausal brain. Harry asks me if I'm OK, if I'm suffering from a touch of jet lag, and I want to tell him the truth: that I think I am losing my mind. That sometimes I worry I am experiencing the early symptoms of Alzheimer's.

I go back to London, hug my daughter, and try to write a piece about Harry that is thoughtful and honest and true. When it is published, I notice that I lose thousands of followers on Instagram.

231

'I'm disappointed that you would collude with such a traitor,' reads one of the more sane missives. 'I feel really let down by you and will be unfollowing immediately.'

'It's an Instagram feed, not an airport,' says Holly, trying to make me feel better. 'No need for everyone to announce their departure.'

I turn off comments on my post, and am flooded with DMs telling me I am a liberal coward stifling free speech.

I feel like I have spent all of 2023 so far in that twilight zone Peter had spoken about.

A week before the coil is due to be fitted, I faint. Humans faint all the time, of course. There are people out there who actually see it as a personality quirk or a party trick, like being able to speak like Donald Duck or touch your nose with your tongue. It's just what they do when they're not working. Sometimes while they *are* working, come to think about it. I used to have a colleague who was prone to faints. That's what she said to me, the first time I saw her collapse, while washing her hands in the office bathroom. 'Oh, don't worry about that!' she said, coming round from her swoon. 'Happens all the time. I'm prone to faints, it's not a problem.'

In common with most people 'prone to faints' she was delicate and dainty, like a little china doll. Needless to say, hulking great big people like me are *not* prone to faints. I have never fainted, not once, not even after taking three grams of cocaine and drinking eighteen pints of Stella. I have the constitution of an ox. I am not a fainter.

But there I am, making breakfast for my daughter, slathering butter on toast, when my heart starts racing at almost 200 beats per minute. I come round on the floor, vaguely grateful that I have fallen on nothing sharper than a butter knife, with my husband peering down at me. 'Doctor,' he demands. 'Now.'

'I'm fine,' I say.

'No, you're fucking not.' He takes my wrist and checks my Apple Watch. 'Your heart is going like the clappers. Seriously, Bryony, you need to get to the GP.'

'I'm sick of doctors, though,' I manage to whinge. 'He'll only tell me I'm being histrionic and doing too much or something. That I need to change my lifestyle, quit my job and concentrate on bringing up a family.'

'He won't say that. Don't be silly.'

'Don't call me silly! I'm not silly!'

I get up and continue making the toast, only with a different knife.

'Bryony, will you please let me do that.' He takes over.

I go upstairs, call the GP, and feel mildly annoyed that I probably won't be able to smoke for the rest of the day.

By a stroke of luck, the surgery finds me an emergency appointment, and I am seen by a female GP who proceeds to take me seriously. She listens to my heart and says it sounds fine, but that to rule out anything more sinister, she wants to book me in for an ECG.

'If this happens again, I want you to promise me that you will go straight to A&E.' She is firm, giving me all her attention. 'At your age, we need to check you're not having a heart attack.'

'I'm not having a heart attack!' I protest. 'I'm just menopausal and stressed!'

'Promise me you'll go to A&E?'

'OK, I promise you.'

I leave, thinking she's being a right drama queen.

When to take your health seriously:

- Always.
- Every day.
- Constantly.
- Even when you think it's 'only' in your head – maybe it is, but better to know that for sure.

The ECG is booked for a week after the coil. My heart stays calm, obedient, as I try to prepare my body for the onslaught of progesterone. I decide that to better handle it, I need to really nurture my body over the next three months. I need to exercise regularly, continue cutting down on caffeine, eat well, and maybe think about giving up smoking.

Gulp.

I read something on Instagram about affirmations, and how they can have a powerful effect on your life. If you say that you are going to have a good day, then you're more likely to. I decide to adopt this approach to things – after all, it can't be any more bonkers than the conversations going on in my head between Jareth, Nigel and Jacob, or the ones in my Instagram comments about the state of the monarchy.

'Good morning, body!' I say when I wake up on the day of the procedure. 'Today we are going to welcome an IUS. It will be moving in with us for the foreseeable future. Let's make it feel as comfortable and at home as possible. If it settles in easily, it's going to make life much easier for all of us.'

'Are you OK?' says Harry, who is half-awake next to me.

'I'm fucking great!' I beam. 'Just getting ready to welcome the coil to my body. Never been happier!'

On the way to the clinic, I surprise my local coffee shop by ordering a decaf.

'Are you OK?' asks the barista, who is used to serving me a caffeinated flat white at least three times a day.

'I'm great!' I beam. 'Never been happier!'

I don't understand why people keep asking me if I'm OK. It's almost as if I'm giving off a slightly manic vibe.

The decaf coffee tastes just like normal coffee, only without the physical kick. That's when I realise: coffee is pointless without caffeine. It tastes *horrible*: acrid and bitter, much like me after you've announced that if I want to live a long and healthy life, I have to stop having fun. It reminds me of the first time I drank non-alcoholic beer, when it quickly became apparent that without the buzz of booze inside it, I was essentially drinking cat's piss.

I'm sure there are people out there who can drink the occasional glass of wine or cup of coffee because they *appreciate the taste*. But I'm not – and never will be – one of them.

'Non-alcoholic drinks are for non-alcoholics,' lectured a rather pious sober person later, when I told them about my experience with pretend beer. 'I stick to water and green juices.'

Is this what my future entails? I think bleakly, as I get on the tube into town. *Water, green juices, fresh air?*

The clinic is in a non-descript building off Oxford Street. It's conveniently located so that you can spend a morning shopping in the giant Primark, before popping round the corner to have an intrauterine device fitted. I ring the bell and a huge man in a black suit answers the door, bearing one of those security passes favoured by bouncers on nightclub doors. I wonder briefly if I have got the wrong building and accidentally stumbled on some secret speakeasy. But then he asks me my name and appointment time, and I notice the woman coming at me from the pavement, clutching a copy of the Bible, and I realise I am in exactly the right place. He's just here to protect patients who might be coming here to have abortions. I say my name loudly, and follow it with the words, 'I'm here to have a coil fitted,' and then I feel a bit ashamed, because I shouldn't feel the need to explain my presence to this woman with a Bible. It's nobody's business what I do with my body, and even if I *was* here to have an abortion, she can bugger off and shove her book where the sun doesn't shine.

He ushers me into the building, shuts the door on Bible Woman, and I think to myself: *What a world we live in. What a fucking world.*

I go down some stairs to a waiting area, where I find a loo and have a pee, noting that decaf coffee has the same effect on my bladder as the real stuff. When I emerge, I am greeted with the sight of a smiling woman in scrubs holding out her hand.

'I'm Edith!' she says, and I am surprised, not having expected to actually meet the woman who had cheered me up so much on the phone. I take her hand and shake it, and she leads me into her office, which isn't really an office, more a mini-operating theatre complete with a bed and various instruments of what I assume to be torture.

Edith sits me down on the bed and asks me how I'm feeling.

'Great!' I lie. 'Never been better.'

'Wonderful,' says Edith, who reminds me of Shirley Ballas, if Shirley Ballas wielded a speculum instead of a paddle bearing various scores for the paso doble.

'So, we're going to start by taking a urine sample to double check you're not pregnant,' she explains.

'I'm definitely not pregnant,' I say. 'And I just went for a wee.'

She hands me a test tube. 'Well, you're going to have to go

for another one. Why don't we get you some water, or perhaps a tea or coffee to help?'

'I don't drink coffee,' I say, because today it's true. I follow her back into reception, get myself a cup of water from the cooler, down it, and then another. In the toilet, I sit and chant positive affirmations. 'My body is ready for this coil,' I say, trying to squeeze out a drip of urine. 'This will be a pain-free and positive experience for me!'

After five minutes trying to coax out a pee, we are able to establish that I am not pregnant (told you so). Edith weighs me, checks my height, and tells me that she thinks body mass index is a terrible way to assess a person's health. She doesn't mention where I land on said index, and I love her a little more for it.

'Right then, sweetheart,' she says, waving a blood-pressure machine in the air. 'Last thing before we get to it.'

My blood pressure is healthy, so we are able to proceed with the coil.

'You could think about it as being similar to having a smear test, only I will provide you with a little local anaesthetic cream,' explains Edith. 'Also, there's a colleague here who can hold your hand while I put it in. Any questions?'

'Yes,' I say. 'Is it true it has strings? And will my husband be able to feel them?'

Edith laughs. 'It's true that the coil has tiny strings to help us when we need to remove it in five years' time. But unless your husband is . . .' She shakes off the thought. 'No, he won't be able to feel them. Now, my love, any more questions?'

'Yes,' I say, nodding. 'Will you be my friend?'

'Ask me again once we've got this procedure out of the way.' She chuckles.

237

I won't go into the full details of how Edith inserts the coil into my womb, other than to say it involves a small amount of swearing (from me).

'Welcome to my woooooooooomb!' I sing at one point, as if I am hosting a strange episode of *MTV Cribs*. I am sore, but weirdly relieved.

Edith tells me she will call in six weeks, but that in the meantime, I should get in touch if I have any problems.

'Not that you're going to have any problems,' she adds. 'It's all going to work out beautifully for you. You're a woman. You've been doing tougher things than this since you were a child, I imagine.'

I go home, crawl into bed, and wait to go mad.

Five minutes pass, and I do not go mad.

Ten minutes pass, and I do not go mad.

Three hours, twenty-five minutes and forty-seven seconds pass, and I do not go mad.

That night, as we get ready for bed, I report to Harry that it has been twelve hours, and I haven't gone mad.

'I mean, I suppose it depends what you mean by "mad"?' he says, once he's finished brushing his teeth.

'I'm sorry about all of this,' I say, sitting on the edge of the bath. 'I've been a dickhead for two and a half years solid.'

'You've been a dickhead for far longer than that, babes,' he says, sitting next to me. 'But you're *my* dickhead.'

'Thanks,' I snort.

'In all seriousness, you haven't been as much of a dickhead as you think you have. I reckon most of the dickheadery takes place in there.' He taps my forehead. 'And you'd be amazed how good you are at hiding that from people. You're far harder on yourself than you need to be.'

238

'Nah, I'm exactly as hard on myself as I need to be.' I stand up, and go to the sink to wash my face. 'I'm an alcoholic with a history of mental illness, and I need to hold myself accountable or it might all go wrong again.'

'Bryony, it's OK for things to go wrong from time to time. It happens. And sometimes, I worry that you're so busy waiting for things to go wrong that you forget to see everything that's right.'

'Maybe,' I concede. 'But that's better than relapsing into a life of misery and madness.'

'You seem pretty miserable right now,' he points out.

'I'm fine, actually. Today, I am fine. And today – and every day – I have to stay vigilant to this stuff. You remember how bad it got when I was in active alcoholism. You know how bad it gets when I have OCD. I can't just put my feet up and relax and hope that I'll stay sober and functioning. I have to do the work! If I don't do the work, I die!'

'The work sounds fucking exhausting,' says Harry. 'Endless therapy, constant twelve-step meetings, way more journalling than is sensible for someone over the age of fourteen, not to mention having to get to the end of the day and list all the ways in which you've sinned and all the people you have to make amends to.'

'You're not an alcoholic; you wouldn't understand.'

'You know you're not just an alcoholic, Bryony? That you're not just mental ill health? You're a load of other things, too. You're great fun and extremely caring and incredibly thoughtful. You're really good at Mario Kart. You're even better at being a mother. And you know all the words to *Hamilton* off by heart. There's not many people who can say that, you know.'

'Lin Manuel Miranda can. He knows all the words to *Hamilton* off by heart.'

'But is he any good at Mario Kart?'

239

'He doesn't need to be!' I squeal. 'He's Lin Manuel Miranda!'

'And you're Bryony fucking Gordon. So try being a bit kinder to yourself.'

I sigh, and storm off into the bedroom, where I can get on with the work of viciously berating myself so that I remain a good, sober alcoholic.

In an attempt to control the uncontrollable, I return to the menopause forums, where I search furiously for the precise amount of time it took for @periperimenopausechick and @fedup to lose their minds after having the IUS fitted.

'Am I the only one who thinks things like IUDs are well dodge?' writes @flowerpowered95. 'Who's to say that the government can't track you through them? Has anyone thought of that?'

'I'm not sure that Rishi Sunak is all that interested in keeping tabs on my vagina,' I begin to type, before deleting the message and thinking that this is actually less outlandish a theory than the plots of some Margaret Atwood books.

'Why is nobody talking about the effects of the vaccine on our reproductive systems?' asks @Beachplea5e. 'I am a healthy, vegan woman in her late forties. I've never drunk, smoked or taken drugs. Everyone says I look ten years younger than I am as a result, lol, and my hubby agrees! Certainly feel like I'm still in my thirties! Then I get the vaccine thinking I am helping society, etc., and almost immediately my periods change, and now my homeopath says that I am going through menopause?? How has nobody made the link between the vaccines and so many women suddenly becoming menopausal??!'

I shut my laptop in despair. It's hard to tell sometimes, whether it's these menopause forums making me feel mad, or the fucking IUS.

*　　*　　*

I faint again a week later.

I get out of bed, and fall back on to it, my eyes rolling back in their sockets, according to Harry.

My heart is off to the races again. I don't tell Harry what the doctor said about calling A&E, because it's the day of my ECG anyway, and if anything is seriously wrong, surely they will pick it up? I recover quite quickly, and decide that the best thing for it is to go for a run. This feels entirely logical to me at the time, like putting wound wash on a cut or placing someone into the recovery position after a seizure.

'I find running meditative,' I tell Harry, as I lace up my shoes. 'It will be good for me. I'll stop if it gets bad again. And anyway, I can run to the health centre for the ECG. They'll be impressed!'

Only a woman could turn a serious medical appointment into an opportunity to people-please.

At the health centre, I sit in the waiting room and feel fairly confident that I am going to be told these episodes are due to panic. To stress. The menopause. I imagine the doctor ordering me to take it easy, perhaps even to take a few weeks off, and to think about making some lifestyle changes – all advice that I will obviously ignore. I think about what a cliché I am, what a drain on NHS resources, given all that I know about panic attacks.

My heart flutters as if in agreement.

Jareth, Nigel and Jacob take the opportunity to chime in.

BG News

Nigel: On today's show, we ask, is Bryony being a massive attention-seeker and time-waster by going to the doctor for an ECG over a little bit of anxiety?

Jacob: Have people like Bryony taken their quest to get everyone talking about mental health issues too far? Are our young people now focusing on their feelings at the expense of thinking about other people? Some might argue that she seems to spend more time worrying about herself than she does her own daughter.

Nigel: Jareth the Goblin King, what are your thoughts?

Jareth: I quite agree, except for one thing.

Nigel: Yes?

Jareth: She's not that young. You referred to 'young people', but she'll be forty-three this year. No spring chicken.

Nigel: She could do with a bit of Botox. Maybe some fillers. I wouldn't shag her.

Jareth: Not even her husband wants to shag her.

Nigel: Can you blame him? Would you want to go to bed with a boring old bat who spends all her time farting on about her issues and problems and how unfair it is to be a woman? From what I've heard, he's been completely emasculated by her. He's a cuckold. He should leave her, get a real woman who looks after herself and cares about her weight and appearance. If I was him, I would have divorced her years ago! What a doormat!

My heart starts up again, perhaps at the realisation that things have gotten *this* bad.

At what stage do I check myself in to the Priory? When Piers Morgan shows up?

I look at the people around me, with real illnesses and prob-lems, and feel guilty. How dare I take up a valuable appointment when I am well enough to *run* here? It's just the menopause! I am only a woman! I am taking up too much space! I am not enough, and too much, all at the same time! If I just lost some weight, complained a little less, and behaved a bit better, none of this would be happening. I make everything more difficult than it needs to be. I cause too much fuss. Other people suffer as a direct consequence of my existing – because of my problems, Harry has to suffer, and Edie has to suffer, and as for my sister and brother and father and mother . . . all they've done for years and years is suffer, suffer, *suffer*.

A doctor calls my name, interrupting my train of thought. Which is more of an express train of doom hurtling towards the apocalypse, really.

I follow the woman to a room where, for the second time in a week, I am to be probed. This time, it's not my womb that is being prodded, but my chest. I am told to take off my top and bra and lie down on the bed. I do as I am told and, as I lie flat on the cold surface, I think I can actually see my heart moving through my skin.

The doctor places a series of sticky circular pads on various parts of my chest and arms, and tells me to relax. She attaches wires to the pads, then sits next to me at a desk, hunched over a black machine that I assume is giving her readings. I look at her, and watch as her face goes from nonchalant to curious to clearly concerned. She realises I am looking at her, and turns to give me a tight smile. Her eyes dart from my face to the screen and back again.

'Are you OK?' she says, her eyes now firmly on whatever the screen is telling her.

'I don't know,' I say, feeling a strange heat rise inside me. 'You tell me.'

'I asked because you're in atrial fibrillation,' she states clearly. 'I'm just making sure I am capturing it right now. Do you have a diagnosis of an arrhythmia?'

'A what?' I am confused, panicky. 'I don't have a diagnosis of anything. I mean, nothing in my heart. Only in my head.'

'OK, Ms Gordon,' she says, pressing some more buttons. 'Please just stay calm and breathe if you can.'

'I can breathe! I am calm!'

'I'm going to need to call an ambulance to take you to A&E.' She picks up the phone next to her, punches in some numbers.

'What? Why? I'm fine. It's just a bit of stress, isn't it?'

'Hi, female, forty-two, in A-Fib,' she says into the receiver. 'Heart hasn't been in sinus rhythm since ECG began. Yep. Yep. Thanks so much.' She puts the phone down. 'Ms Gordon, you're going to need to get dressed now. Can you manage that?' She is talking to me very slowly, as if I am stupid, or unwell. 'The paramedics will be here any minute. I don't want you to panic; you're in safe hands. But protocol states that I can't deal with arrhythmias here at the health centre, so we're going to take you to the hospital. Is there someone you can call?'

I shake my head, unable to speak. And then I burst into tears, like the pathetic woman-child I am.

15

Hysterical

Snapshot from my iPhone's Notes App, January 2023

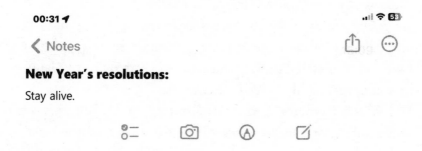

00:31 ⌤   ⊿ 🛜 🔋

‹ Notes   ⬆️ •••

New Year's resolutions:

Stay alive.

☑☰   📷   Ⓐ   ☑️

Later, I will see the timing as divine.

Magic, in a way.

But in this moment, I am simply in shock.

The two paramedics who arrive at the health centre are female. In the past, I might have dismissed this detail as irrelevant, but in light of all my experiences in the last year, I now see it as absolutely central to the fact that I am finally being taken seriously. That I am finally taking *myself* seriously. I think of the random bit of luck that resulted in me being booked in to see a woman when I called the GP's surgery the morning after I fainted. It was her who had insisted that I get an ECG, and who had taken me seriously enough to tell me I should go to A&E if it happened again – something I would never have dreamed of, for fear of being seen as wasting the NHS's time. Had I phoned five minutes earlier or five minutes later, or fainted the day before, would I have ended up with the same male doctor and been dismissed? Might I have walked home from the appointment gaslighting myself for being a drama queen, an attention-seeker?

Clara and Kate swoop into the room in a blizzard of reassuring smiles.

'Now then, Ms Gordon, can you tell me a bit of background?' Clara is my age, South African. I imagine that in another life, we could just as easily be discussing horoscopes together. I feel immediately relaxed around her, and start to tell her how I have found myself sitting in this health centre on a cold January morning, feeling like a bit of a twat.

'I'm a bit embarrassed, truth be told,' I say. 'In that very middle-class, British way where you don't want to be seen to make a fuss, even when you've been told your heart is doing something it shouldn't.'

'Of course you're embarrassed,' says Clara, putting on a blood pressure monitor. 'You're a woman; you've always been dismissed.'

I'm even more embarrassed when I realise that I am crying.

As Clara takes my pulse, she tells me a story about her wife, who went to the doctor because she was experiencing excruciating pain in her stomach and lower back. The GP told her it was probably a bad case of PMS, and sent her home with nothing more than some vague advice to take paracetamol and ibuprofen. The next day, Clara's wife had started to run a fever of almost forty degrees and was unable to move. Being a paramedic, Clara bundled her wife into the car and took her to A&E, where she was diagnosed with a serious kidney infection that required her to stay in for treatment for three days. 'So, you know, we get it.' Clara smiles.

'Yeah.' Kate nods. 'When I went into labour, the hospital told me to go for a walk and call back when "things got really painful",' she says, waggling her fingers in the air in a comic manner. 'I had my son twenty-five minutes later on my kitchen floor, at which point it seemed a little bit too late to call them back.'

'It's our lot.' Clara sighs.

'Did you know that the word "hysteria" comes from the Greek word for uterus?' asks Kate.

'Explains a lot,' says Clara.

'I had to stop working for three years when I turned fifty,' says the woman who did my ECG, speaking up quite suddenly from her desk in the corner. 'I thought I was going mad, but it turned out I was just going through the menopause.'

'*Just* going through a process with dozens of debilitating symptoms that, were it any other condition, would make you assume you were dying,' trills Clara. 'Night sweats, chest pain, memory loss, unbearable hot flashes that feel like you're being boiled alive like a frog! I tell you what' – she pauses to put an oximeter on my finger – 'they've got a lot of bloody cheek calling *us* hysterical.'

*　　*　　*

249

Later, I read up on the gaslighting that women experience in medical settings. Turns out that as well as the gender pay gap, there is also a gender *health* gap. A 2018 study that analysed journal papers about gender and pain found that women were more likely than men to have their experiences dismissed as over-exaggerated or even imaginary, existing only in their heads. The study revealed that terms such as 'sensitive', 'malingering', 'complaining' and 'hysterical' were more frequently attached to pain reports from women. Meanwhile, a 2016 study in the UK found that women were fifty per cent more likely to be misdiagnosed after a heart attack, with the pain often being put down to anxiety. The outcomes are even worse if you are a woman of colour. The Royal College of Obstetricians and Gynaecologists reported in 2020 that Black women experienced many more delayed or even missed diagnoses than white women, especially in maternal and reproductive health.

None of this is surprising, sadly. It wasn't until the 1990s that a law was introduced so that women actually had to be included in medical trials. Until then, men were seen as representative of the entire species, which seems utterly ludicrous given how very different we are on a biological level. The result is that while ninety per cent of women report at least one PMS symptom, there are five times more studies into erectile dysfunction, which affects only nineteen per cent of men.

As Clara might say: Hysterical my *arse*.

Are you being a Mad Woman,
or are you a perfectly reasonable human?

1. A man you have been seeing for two months suddenly ghosts you. You WhatsApp him to tell him that you think this behaviour is rude. Are you:
   A) a Mad Woman?
   B) a perfectly reasonable human?
2. You raise your voice in a work meeting because you haven't been able to get a word in edgeways. Are you:
   A) a Mad Woman?
   B) a perfectly reasonable human?
3. You express emotion when things get on top of you. Are you:
   A) a Mad Woman?
   B) a perfectly reasonable human?
4. You voice your needs to a man without apologising. Are you:
   A) a Mad Woman?
   B) a perfectly reasonable human?
5. You go through a biological process that has an array of exhausting symptoms, both mental and physical, and feel overwhelmed by it. Are you:
   A) a Mad Woman?
   B) a perfectly reasonable human?

If this were a movie, or at the very least a Netflix mini-series, I would obviously be blue-lit to the hospital in an ambulance, sirens wailing and lights flashing, a doctor in scrubs immediately leaping on to my chest to perform compressions as Clara and Kate furiously push the stretcher through to the OR, or whatever it's called in the NHS, where George Clooney or Hugh Laurie or – fingers crossed – Ellen Pompeo from *Grey's Anatomy* would be awaiting me. But because I am absolutely not hysterical or attention-seeking, it's nothing like that. Instead, as befits the magnificent, crumbling, underfunded National Health Service, everything happens very slowly, with Clara and Kate frequently having to hand out the proviso that it might not happen at all.

I am feeling OK by the time I clamber into the back of the ambulance on Clapham High Street. Clara and Kate tell me my heart is now in 'sinus rhythm', which means it isn't trying to escape from my chest like a pterodactyl any more.

A cyclist tuts at us as he passes, because . . . we are taking up space? The ambulance is parked in his cycle lane? We are not thinking about the divine right of the Middle-Aged Man In Lycra trying to smash a PB while cycling through central London? I wonder what it would take for him not to be annoyed by me. Would it be better if I was being pushed into the back of the ambulance on a stretcher with a neck brace on? Or in a body bag? I love many men, and I am aware of how important it is not to generalise, but my experiences over the last few months have left me profoundly aware of the inherent entitlement that seems to run through some of them at times when they could really do with being a little bit more compassionate.

From the ambulance, I call Harry, who seems just as shocked as I am. 'You mean, you *actually* have something wrong with you?' he gasps. 'It's not just your nerves?'

'They say it's a result of being married to you,' I deadpan.

'I will collect Edie from school,' he says, trying to be helpful.

'Just one thing. Well, two, actually. Firstly, what time do I need to be at the school? And secondly, where do I pick her up from?'

'You pick her up from *the school she has been attending for almost six years*. That one. Go up to the gates and tell them that despite looking like a strange man, you are actually the father

252

of one of the children in year five. Go there at 3.20pm. That's twenty past three.'

'And then what?'

'Parent your child?'

'Maybe we should come and sit with you in the hospital?' he suggests, I think genuinely believing himself to be helpful.

'No, no, it's OK,' I insist. 'I wouldn't want to worry Edie, and I'll be fine on my own!'

As the ambulance pulls away, Clara asks if there's any particular artist I'd like to listen to while we make our way to the hospital.

'Taylor Swift, particularly from the *Reputation* era,' I suggest.

Kate high-fives me, and Clara puts on 'Look What You Made Me Do'.

As the song changes to 'I Did Something Bad', I ask Kate a question.

'This . . . atrial fibrillation thing. Did I cause it?'

'Do you know that never, in my seventeen years working as a paramedic, has a man asked me if they *caused* whatever they're in the ambulance for.' Kate smiles. 'Not even the ones who are here because they've got plastered down the pub and ended up in a fight with Big Ron for looking at them dodgy. It's always the women who ask if it's their fault. Do you know the most heartbreaking case I've ever seen?'

I shake my head.

And she tells me a story I am unlikely to ever forget, about arriving to a scene to find a young woman, no more than twenty-five, whose face was completely shattered. Cheekbones broken, eyes black and blue, lips basically torn open. Hair matted with blood. She hadn't called the ambulance, mind you. The police had, and they'd only been called out themselves because the neighbours had dialled 999 after hearing the screams from next door. The young woman had been beaten up by her boyfriend, not that she wanted to make a song and dance about it.

'It was a "domestic".' Kate waggles her fingers in the air again, although this time it doesn't feel quite so amusing. 'I'm always stunned when that word gets used to describe appalling violence. You get called to domestics and other paramedics – men *and* women, I have to say – roll their eyes as if they're annoyed to be having to help someone who has been beaten half to death by the father of her children. As if they'd have preferred it if she had just capitulated to him, been a good girl, not done whatever it is that's prompted him to use his fists. Anyway, this woman does *not* want an ambulance, let alone the police. She's sitting on the floor of the living room, blood all around her on the carpet, and she's screaming, half in pain and half because she knows that us being there is only going to make matters worse later. She knows she's going to be made to come to the hospital with us and that we will try to comfort her, tell her that she's safe now. But she also knows that, in all likelihood, she's not safe at all. She's going to get cleaned up, stitched up, sent home, and she's not going to press charges because she's in an abusive relationship and she's worn down and she's scared, and as soon as he gets home from the police station, she's going to be treading on eggshells, keeping herself small so she doesn't provoke him into beating her again.'

I sit quietly. The tale is all too familiar.

'Anyway, we manage to get her into the ambulance. And on the way there, do you know what she says to me? She says, "It's my fault. I shouldn't have gone out with my friends when he asked me not to." She wasn't having it that she might be entitled to exist without him driving his knuckles into her face.'

254

The Taylor Swift song has gone quiet. There is nothing more to say.

At the hospital, I hug Clara and Kate, and am taken to a cubicle, where a nurse tells me I will need to have yet another ECG, as well as having some bloods done. There is a junior doctor's strike on, which means the average waiting time is eight hours. I'd assumed that was about the average waiting time when there wasn't a strike on, so I am almost impressed by the brevity. Also, I'm not going to lie: I'm kind of looking forward to a day of lying down in a cubicle with nothing but my dodgy heart for company. To be excused from the daily burden of meeting eighteen different deadlines in time to pick my child up from school is the kind of luxury I haven't experienced since I went into labour with her (and even then, I had to sit on a birthing ball with my laptop propped on my thighs, filing columns to ensure I was ahead by the time she arrived two days later). The nurse apologises about the wait; I tell him he doesn't have to worry.

I've got a lot to think about.

Paul, for example. An early boyfriend of mine, whose parting words to me were that nobody would ever love me the way he did. This love of his involved bruises and rage and jewellery ripped from my throat and always, always, the sense that it would be different if maybe I was less erratic, if perhaps I was less mad, if I was cooler and calmer and less prone to winding him up.

I think about the man who pursued me so relentlessly that in the end, I agreed to go on a date with him because that seemed easier than getting a restraining order. I think about the sex that I went through with because I didn't want him to think I was a prick tease; fingers inserted into bits of me that I hadn't asked for or agreed to. I think about how, afterwards, I actually made

255

a joke of it to friends, because even as recently as the noughties, it was just easier to do this.

I think about all the men who have written to me to tell me I am fat and ugly and that they wouldn't want to have sex with me if I was the last woman on earth – giving me answers to questions I hadn't even asked in the first place.

I think about Michael, too. Married. Far more senior than me in the industry. The man I allowed to treat me like a worthless piece of shit, because that was exactly what I thought I was. The man who told me, when I suggested that we do something for my thirtieth birthday, that I was 'just sex' to him. I think about how I went back two weeks later, for more. Because I thought I could change his mind. I thought if I made him love me, it would all be better.

I think about how these experiences are not even that unusual. That they are pretty ordinary snapshots from the lives of many women my age.

And I think that the worst thing about all of this is that I colluded with so many of these men. I thought so little of myself that it didn't occur to me to protect myself from them, or speak out against them. And when they were gone, having moved on to the next woman, I actually pined for them, and agonised over what it was *I* had done wrong.

No, that's not the worst thing.

The worst thing is the voice in my head accusing me of playing the victim.

Urggggh.

Conversations with my mother: Part four

I call my mum, because that's what you do when you unexpectedly find yourself in hospital, even if you are in your forties.

'I'm just about to take the dog for a walk with Kerry, can I call you back?' she says, hurriedly.

'Actually Mum, I'm in hospital.'

'You're WHAT?'

'I'm in hospital, I've got some sort of heart thing.'

'I'm leaving the dog with Kerry and coming NOW. Don't try and stop me! I'm getting into the car right this minute!'

'It's OK, Mum, you don't have to—'

'I bloody do have to, I'm your mum! What's happening?'

'I've been having these palpitations, and it turns out that I have some sort of atrial fibrillation thing. You don't need to worry, I'm fine, it's just I wanted to call you and tell you and . . . and I don't know what, really.'

'I knew there was something up with you. You've not been yourself recently. All these questions about the menopause. The stress of the pandemic. You need your mum! I can be with you in five minutes.'

'You live a two-hour drive away.'

'I know, but maternal anxiety will speed me up.'

'It's really OK. I would much rather you stayed where you are and just chatted to me while I wait here at the hospital.'

'Can you tell me what happened?'

I tell her about the palpitations and the ECG and the paramedics.

'I'm so proud of you,' she says, suddenly.

'What?'

'You sound so calm, so measured. You were such an anxious

257

child, but you've grown into such a remarkable woman. Even when you're in hospital with a heart thing, you exude this sort of . . . *serenity.*'

'I'm not so sure about—'

'The thing about your generation, Bryony, is you have a *chance.* I used to think that meant you had a chance to smash through glass ceilings and have it all, but actually you have a chance to take yourselves seriously. To not dismiss yourselves simply because you happened to have been born with two X chromosomes. I'm so glad that you got yourself to the doctor and are getting proper care. I'm so glad you took yourself seriously. I'm so glad they took you seriously. I think it's about time, don't you, that us women were allowed to take ourselves seriously?'

Bloods are taken, another ECG is carried out. The nurse fits me with a Holter monitor, which will record my heart rate for three days, giving doctors a better picture of what it's actually doing. Eventually, a specialist arrythmia nurse arrives to speak to me. His name is Steve. He is calm and softly spoken, one of the many good men I need to remember I encounter each and every day.

'So, how are you feeling?' he asks, sitting down in the chair next to my bed.

'Oh, you know. Just relieved I don't seem to be dying of a heart attack. But not really sure what *is* going on.'

'OK, well your heart was in atrial fibrillation for quite a long time this morning,' he explains. 'Atrial fibrillation happens when the top chambers of your heart beat out of time with the other chambers.' He forms his hands into something vaguely resembling a heart to try and demonstrate what has been going on in my chest. 'For any number of reasons, the top chamber starts to quiver and twitch. It's not deadly. It won't kill you. It's uncomfortable, of course, especially if you are in it constantly, but you seem to be back in sinus rhythm now, which means we would refer to you as having paroxysmal atrial fibrillation.'

I raise my eyebrows to display how impressed I am by the exotic sound of this condition.

'I know it's a lot to take on, so tell me to stop if you need to ask any questions.'

I nod at him to continue.

'So the thing about A-Fib is that while it isn't dangerous in itself, people who have it are about five times more at risk of stroke than people without it. That's because when the heart doesn't pump properly, there's a danger of blood clots forming. These clots can move into the lower chambers of the heart and then get pumped into the blood supply to the lungs, or just the blood circulation generally. And those clots can block arteries in the brain, causing a stroke.'

'Oh,' I say, because I'm unsure of what else there is *to* say.

'Because of your age and your blood-pressure readings, we've calculated that your stroke risk is very low, so we don't need to give you blood thinners. But I'm going to prescribe you some beta-blockers that I want you to keep on you at all times. If you think you are going into A-Fib, you take one and it will help you return to sinus rhythm. Does that make sense?'

'It makes as much sense as I could hope, given that this morning I thought I was being overdramatic and now I learn that I actually have a legitimate heart condition.'

'Any questions?'

'So many,' I say. 'For a start, why have I got this?'

'We don't know. It's quite common, more so in the elderly, but young people get it, too. We will get you booked in for an echocardiogram, which will scan your heart and allow us to see what's going on.'

Though he has told me A-Fib won't kill me, my brain has already begun its frantic questioning about other things that might.

'Is it possible I have heart disease?' I say. 'Caused by binge eating chorizo?'

Steve narrows his eyes, perhaps in confusion. 'It *can* be caused by heart disease, but your blood readings don't suggest that's the case. As I said, the echocardiogram will tell us more.'

'Is it because of stress? Or the menopause?'

'It could be because of any number of things,' he says. 'The biggest risk factors are drinking heavily and diabetes.'

'I'm sober,' I tell him a little too keenly. 'I used to drink heavily, but I haven't done for almost six years.'

'Well then, it won't have been caused by that.'

'Is there anything else I can do to help it?'

'It says here that you smoke,' says Steve, looking at his notes. 'If you can, I would try and give up, and if that sounds too hard, at least cut down. Also, caffeine can trigger it, so if you could cut back on that . . .'

'Always with the smoking and the caffeine,' I sigh. '*Always* with the smoking and the caffeine.'

16

Still small voice

Snapshot from my iPhone's Notes App, February 2023

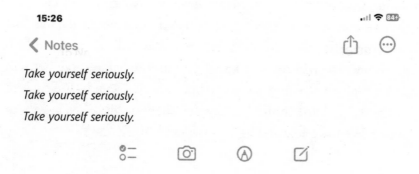

Take yourself seriously.
Take yourself seriously.
Take yourself seriously.

In my twenties, I thought I would live forever. I thought that the rules that applied to older people didn't apply to me. I could smoke and drink and take drugs, because I was young and there was only this moment. Tomorrow didn't matter, because tomorrow wasn't now, and now was almost always too painful or anxiety-inducing for me to just sit back and wait for it to pass. But as I stand in a queue at the hospital pharmacy, waiting to collect my prescription for beta-blockers, I know that the time has finally come to grow the fuck up. To stop burying my head in the sand, because the sand has started to fill my nostrils and my mouth, and is now beginning to suffocate me.

There are all sorts of qualities about addicts that make us annoying and frustrating and frankly unliveable with. We do terrible things to ourselves (and, inadvertently, to others) because they briefly give us relief from pain, even if in the long run they only cause more of it. We are told again and again that if we continue to behave in the way we are, we will harm ourselves, and yet we usually have to wait until we are three minutes away from death before we will even consider stopping said behaviours. We lie and we cheat, and we cause upset and harm to others. We are all the bad things people say we are, and often even worse.

But if you get us in recovery, we are also kind and compassionate and wise. We will give you our time when it feels like everyone else has given up on you. We will sit and we will listen and we will let you know you are not alone. We get shit done. We've got sober, so everything else is a cinch. We look at unspeakably hard things and we see them as gifts. We see them glitter. We have learned to pan for gold in the dark.

The best things about addicts (in recovery)

- We are tenacious.
- We don't judge.
- We've been there, done that and got the T-shirt.

- You can tell us anything.
- We rise to a challenge.
- We have a high tolerance for stress.
- We will always say sorry.
- We will always help with the washing-up.

And so, as I stand in the queue for my medicine, I know immediately what I have to do. I have to change, again. Me, my heart condition and my week-old coil – we are going to have to adapt to the circumstances in which we find ourselves. You won't see cool things if you don't keep moving. And I know enough about addiction to realise that, in being diagnosed with a heart condition, I have been given an opportunity. An opportunity to quit smoking and caffeine, and try to build up the self-esteem I seem to have thrown away in the last two and a bit years. Because when you hit rock bottom, there's only one way out. Actually, there are two ways out, but there's only one way that I *want* to take, and that's up.

If I walk out of this hospital and light up a cigarette, then the only way I am going to stop smoking is if I drop dead of a heart attack. So as much as I think I deserve some sort of treat that is actually a poisonous death sentence, I also know that I have smoked my last cigarette. I am an ex-smoker. There is no turning back, and I am kind of relieved.

Because every time I smoked, every time I binged, every time I had another double espresso that I knew was going to give me the jitters, a still small voice in my head told me that it was a bad idea, that by having a cigarette or bingeing on sausages or drinking so much caffeine I was practically in an altered state, I was harming myself. This Still Small Voice is not Jareth or Nigel or Jacob, and it is not the Stay Puft Marshmallow Man, or any of the other names I have given to the viciously critical chatter that seems to fill my brain. This Still Small Voice wishes me no harm, bears me no ill, wants only the best for me. And that's because this Still Small Voice is my soul.

Does that sound cheesy? Do I even care? I feel as if I have been saved by what has happened today. I think about how our souls are always speaking to us; it's just that some of us are better at hearing them than others. In the past, there have been moments when I have listened, when I have stayed still and quietened the noise of Jareth for long enough to be able to take in what was being said by my soul. When I wrote *Mad Girl*, even though I was told that writing about my type of OCD was inappropriate, I was listening to my soul. When I set up Mental Health Mates, even though I was in the midst of a breakdown and already had a full-time job, I was listening to my soul. When I decided to run that marathon in my pants, even though I was a size twenty and it was entirely possible everyone would laugh at me, I was listening to my soul. When I took myself to rehab, even though I couldn't actually afford it and I had a book deadline to meet, I was listening to my soul.

But for the last few years, I have not been listening to my soul.

I have been listening to Jareth. Jareth, who can shape-shift endlessly, from Nigel to Jacob to the Stay Puft Marshmallow Man, but who is most terrifying of all when I mistake his voice for my own. Jareth, who I stupidly thought I had somehow beaten because of my sobriety, but who I now realise is as addictive to me as any drink, drug, cigarette or item of food. Jareth, who has lived in my brain for so long that I often don't know where I end and he begins. Jareth, who is in direct opposition to the Still Small Voice that is my soul, even if he wants to tell me that he is there to help protect it.

What Jareth says

vs

What the Still Small Voice would say

'You're a lazy, good-for-nothing bum.'

You need to rest, my love.

'That person hates you.'

Hate is a pretty strong word – and if that person does dislike you, then that's their issue.

'You're about to be sacked.'

If your employer has a problem with you, it is their responsibility to tell you and make things better.

'You're useless.'

You're a normal human being who makes the usual mistakes, like everyone else.

I pick up the medicine and decide I am going to take a taxi home. I start to berate myself for being wasteful and profligate, and then I realise that talking to myself like this achieves nothing. It helps no one. I go ahead and order an Uber, and as I sit in the back, I think about all the times I have drowned out the Still Small Voice, with the binge eating and the self-loathing and the airtime I have afforded Jareth.

Has my soul had to resort to making my heart beat like an escaping pterodactyl to get my attention?

If so, she can rest assured.

Finally, I am listening.

17

Heartwork

Snapshot from my iPhone Notes App, March 2023

It's time to wake up, Bryony.
You no longer have the option to keep snoozing your cosmic alarm clock.

An echocardiogram is a bit like the ultrasound scans I had when I was pregnant with Edie, except the doctor smears jelly over your chest instead of your stomach, and then you lie there with your boobs flopping to the side like deflated bean bags as they move the small probe around and tell you about the triathlon they've just completed in Spain.

271

I mean, I can't promise you that this is what *every* echocardiogram is like, but it's certainly an accurate description of the one I have.

'How was your weekend?' the doctor asks, as I lie there, wondering when I will have a hospital appointment that doesn't involve my boobs migrating towards my knees.

'It was fine, thank you,' I reply politely, reasoning that there is no need to tell him about my trip to Sainsbury's, or the visit to John Lewis to finally buy that fucking Bosch tumble dryer, three full years after my husband and I first started discussing it. 'How was yours?'

'Well, I just got back from a big weekend in Marbella. *Big* weekend, you know?' He stares directly at the screen in front of him, where my heart beats in grey like a big, bouncing baby. He hasn't looked me in the face once, perhaps because I am naked from the waist up, perhaps because I am just work to him. Fair enough.

'Oh yes?' I say, taking the bait.

'Well I did a triathlon, you know.' He pretends to be coy, embarrassed.

I decide to play along with him, to make the whole experience a little less awkward. He is, after all, moving a plastic probe back and forth between my naked tits.

'Oh wow,' I say. 'Tell me more.'

'Well, a triathlon is really hard, you know?'

I nod along, sure he is about to mansplain exercise to me.

'I wasn't sure I would be able to do it. You have to swim in the sea, then get on a bike, and then run, all for a really long time. It's kind of mad. Like, normally, you'd only do *one* of those things, but in a triathlon you have to do all three.'

I wonder if he thinks that as well as having a dodgy heart, I only have half a brain.

'Gosh.' I smile.

'It was really hot, you know? But we totally smashed it. So I'm feeling pretty proud of myself today. Ironman next!'

He carries on swishing the probe around my chest while staring directly at the screen in front of him.

'I've done a triathlon,' I say, after a minute or so of silence.

For the first time, he turns away from the screen and looks directly at me. He looks . . . surprised.

'You have?'

'Yeah. Mostly I remember being kind of embarrassed by the stupid triathlon outfit I had to wear through it all. Never trust an outfit designed for swimming, cycling *and* running!'

'I hope you at least happened to do it somewhere cooler than Marbella,' he says. 'The heat made it EXTRA awful, I think.'

'It was in Sardinia, actually,' I state.

'Well, good for you.' He turns back to the screen. 'What prompted you to do it?'

'Probably the same thing that prompted you,' I reply. 'I like a challenge. Like to get out of my comfort zone.'

I allow a polite smile to settle on my face.

'So do you do much exercise, then?' he asks.

'Oh yes.' I nod. 'I've done two marathons. A couple of dozen half marathons. Last year I did ten ten-kilometre runs in ten days to raise money for Mental Health Mates, the not-for-profit organisation I set up seven years ago.'

'Well, well.' He starts to chuckle. 'How extraordinary. How utterly extraordinary.' He removes the probe from my chest. 'I'm all done here. Lovely to meet such an accomplished athlete.'

'And you,' I say, pulling my robe over my naked breasts and standing up.

I get dressed behind a curtain. I don't bother to shake his hand on the way out.

There is nothing wrong with my heart.

That's what Steve the arrhythmia nurse tells me when he calls a couple of days later.

'Structurally, your heart is perfectly healthy,' he says. 'There's no heart disease or anything like that causing the atrial fibrillation. We refer to this as "idiopathic" A-Fib, which means that there's no obvious reason for it. It happens spontaneously. It's far more common than you'd think.'

'So you don't know what caused it?'

'It's possible that a combination of lots of things has led to your episodes of A-Fib. But the good news is that we've ruled out any of the more serious causes. We're going to keep an eye on it. We'll book you back in for an appointment in three months to see how you're getting on, OK?'

'OK.'

'And in the meantime, if you have any problems, you're to call me. Do you have any other questions?'

'It's not really a question,' I reply. 'It's more that I wanted to tell you that I gave up smoking. And caffeine.'

'You did?' He sounds genuinely delighted. 'How long has it been?'

'I haven't had a cigarette since I left the hospital that day. So, a month. Oh, and I've only had decaf.'

'That's bloody brilliant,' he says. 'How do you feel?'

'I mean, annoyingly, a million times better. Turns out that coffee is basically panic juice for me, and that not smoking means I have way more energy. Who knew?' I laugh. 'Actually, don't answer that. Everyone knew.'

Holly sends me a link to a podcast she thinks I should listen to. 'DO NOT ROLL YOUR EYES AT THIS,' she writes in the text accompanying the link. 'Just trust me and listen to it. OK?'

The podcast features a man called Dr Roger Teel. Dr Roger Teel describes himself as a 'life-transforming speaker, a gifted community builder, and a global spiritual leader.'

This is enough for me to call Holly and check that she's OK.

'Holl, please tell me you are not asking me to listen to a pod-cast by a' – I squint as I look closer at the screen in front of me, which is displaying his website – '*church minister from Oregon.*'

'Bryony, church ministers from Oregon are people too.'

'Yes, but they're not *our* people.'

'How would you know, though?' she replies, not entirely unreasonably. 'You're dismissing this dude without listening to him. How do you know that your destiny isn't to pack up your life in south London and move to Oregon to worship at the altar of the gifted community builder Dr Roger Teel?'

'I thought you knew me Holly.' I snigger. 'But now I'm begin-ning to question your judgement. Let me read you some extracts from his website.'

'You don't need to.'

'Oh, I do.' I put on the world's worst American accent. '"As a young child, gazing into the sunlit sky, Roger experienced a mystical awareness of the Oneness of all Life, a knowing that stayed with him throughout his growing years."'

'Bryony,' snaps Holly. 'I would suggest that right now, cynicism is a luxury you don't have. You've been stuck in a depression for god knows how long—'

'I haven't been in a depression,' I say defensively. 'I know what depression is. I've just been behaving like a bit of a dickhead.'

'That's the depression speaking,' Holly sighs. 'Instead of

listening to it, or Jareth, or the Stay Puft Marshmallow Man, or whatever it is you call the negative voices in your head, may I suggest you listen to Dr Roger Teel instead? He does at least have the advantage of being real. You might even learn something.'

She puts the phone down.

I only put the podcast on so she'll speak to me again.

Podcasts for men vs Podcasts for women

For men: An inconsequential man interviews another inconsequential man about how living a keto lifestyle enabled them to take over the world.

For women: An incredibly accomplished woman interviews another incredibly accomplished woman about all the times they fucked up.

I go for a run, because if I'm going to have to listen to Roger, then I may as well spend the time doing something useful.

It is one of the first vaguely warm days of 2023. Spring is undoubtedly in the air. This annoys me, because I really don't want my life to seem like a GCSE English project about pathetic fallacy, and yet this feels like the direction it is generally going in: protagonist experiences run of difficulties that leave her at rock bottom in the winter, and is forced to turn a corner when her much wiser friend makes her listen to the words of a global spiritual leader called Roger, just as the sun breaks through the clouds for spring.

I head towards Battersea Park, because the podcast is over an hour long, and if I'm going to listen to it I'm going to need to travel a distance that is out of my usual comfort zone (within 400 metres of my house).

My first surprise is that running doesn't feel too gloopy. Too awful. I'm almost . . . enjoying it? My second is that Roger is actually quite a jolly fellow, not at all cultish or sinister. He doesn't want me to join his ministry; he just wants me to feel joy. Pure, unadulterated joy. He tells me that I can feel joy even in grief, through realising the love I have for the person I am grieving. He says that nothing outside myself will help me access my joy. He says that to do that, I have to open my heart.

My heart.

'Your spiritual heart and your physical heart are deeply connected,' he says. 'The heart is truly the most intelligent and powerful aspect of our lives. We are discovering that, actually, your heart centre is far more intelligent than your brain.'

I stop at the traffic lights just outside the park, wait for the green man, listen to Roger as he speaks.

'The heart in you and me can be the portal into a deep, lasting joy,' he says. 'Sometimes we have to go through the deepest challenges of our lives to discover our hearts.'

I cross the road into the park, picking up the pace so I am running quite hard and quite fast for me. My blood pumps, my heart beats, feeling strong for the first time since those 10Ks last year. I listen as Roger tells me about the time he had his heart broken. He was about to get engaged to a woman he had been with for four years. They spent Christmas together. One morning, he woke up and found a note from her, saying she never wanted to see him again. She had taken all her things and left.

'And I had to go through the deep grieving, and the confusion,' he says, straight to me. 'I went into the resentment and bitterness and even hating her. I was really descending into a very perilous and difficult place.'

I realise I am by the great big gold Buddha that overlooks the River Thames, the one I had always thought of as utterly arbitrary and frankly a little bit pointless, given that so much of the gold has been scratched away by south London teenagers graffitiing their love for one another on the base of his peace pagoda.

'There's a part of life that is here to help every one of us,' says Roger. 'And I just pause to invite you to know that there are forces around you that are seeking to help you all the time. All you gotta do is ask. And I asked. I got so miserable that I asked. And then a number of realisations started coming to me. The first realisation was that the relationship [with the woman who left] wasn't authentic, and I didn't want to look at it. But the other realisation that came as I kept working with this, was that this betrayal, this *wounding*, was actually calling me to open my heart.'

I sit down on the steps below the Buddha, looking up at the bright blue sky and the seagulls circling in it. I listen to Roger, and I think of him sitting there in Oregon in his church, getting so miserable that he asked . . . for help, for guidance, for the ability to look inside, when it is so much easier and more accepted to blame everything on the issues *outside* of you.

'I had gone through an early portion of my life with a protected and closed heart. And we do this because of fear. That was the key. I spent several years doing deep, intense work to open my heart, and that's when I reconnected with deep joy. I believe that, more than anything else, we are centres of love and light. We are here to express that love, and any time we fall into fear-based living and close our hearts, we distance ourselves from our power. We distance ourselves from joy. We distance ourselves from all the good of life.'

OK, so it's a bit cloying. But it's so much better than listening to Jareth and his demented friends on BG News.

'I'm going to invite you to understand that there is a connection between your heart and its openness, and the depth of the joy you feel. You can reconnect with this joy by being willing to relax into, and open, your heart. I have found that it's usually our own sense of worthiness that we have to take a look at. It's being willing to open our own hearts, and love ourselves first of all.'

I realise, with genuine surprise, that I am not rolling my eyes, but smiling with them.

'I want to give you a gift,' says Roger. 'It's a declaration that can be very powerful in opening the heart. It can be very powerful in healing.' He explains it is a quote from the author and motivational speaker Leo Buscaglia, who was famous in the eighties for seeking to find the answer to human disconnectedness. Roger suggests that everyone listening writes the Buscaglia quote on a piece of paper, to read to themselves when they are in distress. I don't have any paper on me, so the Notes app on my iPhone will have to do. I start typing as Roger speaks, noting down the words that come out of his mouth.

I will love you no matter what.
I will love you if you are stupid, if you slip and fall on your face, if you do the wrong thing, if you make mistakes, if you behave like a human being.
I will love you no matter what.

I text Holly the broken heart emoji. And, just to lighten the mood, the word 'oof'.

Chicken soup for the cynical soul (a recipe)

Ingredients

- A mixture of hippy-dippy New Age books and podcasts about spirituality or some such.
- One cup of open-mindedness.
- One tablespoon of self-awareness.
- 500g of the ability to see that you have no right to judge people who believe in God when, until recently, you only believed in your inalienable right to get shit-faced.
- 250ml of willingness to learn something new.
- A pinch of the possibility that you are sometimes wrong about things.

Method

Use a whisk to mix everything together in a bowl. Leave for a few hours and see what happens. You will be surprised by how good it makes you feel! Repeat daily, until you experience spiritual awakening/entire psychic change.

Like most little girls, I learned that I had to be good. That if I was to please my parents and my grandparents and my teachers, I needed to behave well. I could not be bad. If I was bad, I would disappoint everyone. Except I *was* bad. I was bad because I ate the Herta frankfurters, and I was bad because I had AIDS, and I was bad because thoughts popped into my head that shouldn't, and I was bad because I took up space that my sister and my brother needed but that I couldn't let them have. Because I was bad.

I was bad, bad, bad.

I have this memory of a session with Peter just before the pandemic, where we talked about the purpose of OCD, the roles it might play for different people.

'Has it ever occurred to you that OCD actually made your life easier when you were a child?' he asked. I couldn't understand what he was talking about. I couldn't understand how he could say that. It only made my life miserable.

'Maybe OCD was your brain's way of trying to keep you safe,' he continued. 'If you had Jareth there, checking every thought for evidence of badness, then you wouldn't actually *be* bad. You could be good through the power of hypervigilance. If you were on high alert the whole time for incoming badness, then you could stop it before it got too far.'

I wasn't entirely sure what he meant.

But now I am.

Now I fucking am.

Why it's OK to sometimes behave badly

- Because that's what humans do.
- Because we don't live in the fucking Marvel universe where people are either superheroes or evil villains.
- Because the role of the Angel Gabriel was only supposed to last for the fifteen minutes of your nursery nativity.
- Because the people who *always* behave badly don't actually give a shit.

281

For the first time in my life – all forty-two and a half years of it – I allow myself to consider the possibility that I might be able to accept *all* of me.

Not just the good bits. Not just the awards and the bestselling books and the podcasts and the celebrity plaudits and the social media followers and the years and months and days of sobriety, and all the other things that I have strived so hard for to make up for my inherent badness.

All of me.

The good, the bad, and the whole heap of humanity that lies somewhere in between.

The frankfurter eating. The imaginary aliens I thought might burst out of my chest. The little girl who thought she had AIDS and that there was going to be a nuclear war. The child who took up all of her mother's energy because, fucking hell, she was really unwell. Really, really unwell. The person whose hair fell out because she was so afraid that she might be a serial-killing paedophile; the teenager who would shove her fingers down her throat and force up her food into the toilet to make herself more attractive, more acceptable, because if boys liked her, then everything would be better, wouldn't it?

The girl who was difficult and tricky and sometimes unpleasant because she was a human.

The twenty-something who loved cocaine and alcohol because she thought it made people like her more, even though the opposite was true; the person who hurt women she didn't know by sleeping with their husbands; the feckless idiot who was late to work and late to deadlines and pissed off editors; the manip-ulative bitch who stole her mother and father's peace of mind and sometimes their money; the lost soul who lied and cheated and behaved like an absolute arsehole.

The thirty-something who couldn't even let her happy-ever-after make her happy, who had to test her lovely husband who'd been sent to her by the universe to finally settle her down and make her *good*. The pregnant woman who was referred to mental health services because of how seriously unwell she became, the progesterone pumping through her at its highest levels yet. The new mother who couldn't stop drinking and drugging, even with a precious baby in her life; the mum who washed up in rehab the day before her daughter started school; the one who, even after all that help and privilege, still managed to get lost in binge eating disorder.

The big, big part of me that I now see *has* been in a depression; the bits of me that berate and flagellate and do bloody good impressions of right-wing television commentators.

All of me.

Even Jareth.

It's the first time I allow myself to believe the possibility that all these random bits of me that make no sense, and perhaps never will, are just what I have had to go through to get where I am today.

Which is sitting on the steps of a desecrated Buddha statue in south London, listening to a Christian minister in Oregon tell me to open my heart.

I mean, listen, I'm an addict. I've been to far worse places.

18

Woo-woo

Snapshot from my iPhone Notes App, April 2023

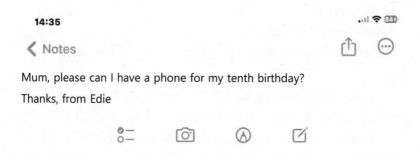

14:35
Notes

Mum, please can I have a phone for my tenth birthday?
Thanks, from Edie

The GCSE project in pathetic fallacy continues. The days get brighter, my heart opens a little further.

I ask Holly to send me some more of her podcast suggestions.

'The woo-woo ones,' I say, with a laugh.

'The way of the woo is the way forward,' says Holly.

'Do you think that the reason women are more likely to be woo-woo than men is because we have been let down by the more traditional systems that are historically patriarchal in nature?'

'I think you're picking up the way of the woo pretty damn quickly, coming out with a sentence like that,' says Holly. 'But I also know that Roger isn't a woman, and he's pretty damn woo-woo.'

'Open your heart!' I say in the world's worst American accent.

'Connect to deep joy!' mimics Holly.

I tune out BG News and Fuckwittery FM and tune in to the Still Small Voice. I tell Holly my theory about said Still Small Voice being my soul, and how I feel that in coining the term, I am destined to be a great spiritual leader, perhaps even greater than Rog, as I've taken to calling him.

Holly grimaces, but in a very polite way.

'Um, I hate to break it to you, babes, but you didn't come up with that term.'

I look at her blankly.

'Don't tell me some wellbeing influencer got there first,' I screech.

'I mean, you could argue that the *ultimate* wellbeing influencer got there first,' she says, shaking her head in what I think might be ... disbelief. 'That phrase is literally in the Bible. It's used to describe the voice of God.'

I shrug, trying to hide my embarrassment. 'I've never read the Bible,' I say, truthfully. 'I'm more into ... Brené Brown.'

'You once told me you'd rather die than become the kind of person who reads Brené Brown.' She's referring to a phase of my life, shortly after we got sober, when I was determined not to lose my old cynical self in all the twelve-step chat about 'higher powers' and so on.

'Well, just watch as I become the kind of person who admits

that I was wrong. It's called getting humble, Holly,' I say, some-what smugly. 'It's called *humility.*'

BG NEWS SPECIAL BULLETIN

Jacob Rees-Mogg: We interrupt our regular programming to bring you some devastating news.

Nigel Farage: It gives us no pleasure to have to tell you this, but as of today, we have been informed that we are to cease broadcasting. Jareth, can you tell us more about what has happened?

Jareth *(spinning his crystal balls)*: Sure, Nigel. So, as you know, it was always a possibility that Bryony would assert her will and stop listening to us. It's happened before, and sadly, it has happened again. I have been given notice that the Still Small Voice I thought we had managed to drown out is coming to close us down.

Nigel: You mean the Still Small Voice of the Wokerati?

Jacob: Actually, the Still Small Voice is more like Ofcom, only for brains.

Nigel: Whose side are you on, spoddy?

Jacob: Well, if you are going to talk to me like *that,* I think you'll find I'm on the side of the Still Small Voice.

Still Small Voice: Guys, it's not that I want to shut you down. If you'd been a bit more balanced and provided some impartial reporting, perhaps this wouldn't have had to happen. But the ratings are down, and Bryony is no longer tuning in. I'm sorry. It's time for something new. Cheerio!

Cut to picture of Test Card Girl, except without the creepy clown.

In an attempt to listen to the Still Small Voice of my soul – not the Still Small Voice of God, just to be clear – I read Brené Brown. *All* of Brené Brown. Every last word she's ever written. I try to imagine what Brené would say to Jareth, were she ever to come across him in her brain. Probably something cool like: 'Dare greatly, have the courage to be vulnerable – and, by the way, nice hair.'

When I have finished with Brené Brown, I move on to Louise Hay, who believes that you can improve your life by staring in the mirror and chanting affirmations to yourself.

'For the next month,' writes Hay in her book *You Can Heal Your Life*, 'say over and over to yourself, "I APPROVE OF MYSELF". Do this three or four hundred times a day, at least. No, it's not too many times. When you are worrying, you go over your problem at least that many times. Let "I approve of myself" become a walking mantra, something you just say over and over to yourself, almost nonstop . . . no matter what happens, no matter who says what to you, just keep it going. In fact, when you can say that to yourself when someone is doing something you don't approve of, you will know you are growing and changing.'

I screw up my face in horror at the idea of having to say 'I approve of myself' 400 times a day. It is as if Louise Hay has read my mind. 'Thoughts have no power over us unless we give in to them,' she continues. 'Thoughts are only words strung together. They have NO MEANING WHATSOEVER. Only *we* give meaning to them. Let us choose to think thoughts that nourish and support us.'

Woo-woo vs Wellness fad

Woo-woo	Wellness fad
Makes you feel uplifted and hopeful	Makes you feel like you need to lose weight
Is free or reasonably priced to cover materials and labour	Requires a loan
Allows you to be yourself	Promises to make you better
Is practised by all kinds of people	Is practised only by people in yoga leggings that cost £150

I google 'strength-training fitness near me' and am immediately directed to a local gym that provides something called 'CrossFit'. CrossFit promises that it is totally inclusive and for all ages and abilities, and that it comes complete with an amazing community. I imagine bake sales and cups of tea, and sign up for my free trial class.

I am shocked to discover that instead of those innocent looking cross-training machines that I had somehow imagined, CrossFit involves Olympic weightlifting, pull-ups, burpees and all other manner of hellish things.

'I approve of myself, I approve of myself, I APPROVE OF MYSELF!' I shout as I do my twenty-seventh burpee of the morning.

When it finally finishes, I realise I am deliriously happy, for the first time in three years.

I sign up for a full membership.

I continue in my quest to read every self-help book ever written. I realise that obsessively filling my brain with texts on mind-fulness and positivity might have seemed trivial to a previous version of me, but to this version, it is almost a matter of life and death. I feel as if my brain is a big lake that I have allowed OCD, depression and binge eating disorder to poison; now I need to clean it, so that life can bloom again inside. I read books by Buddhist monks, books by Buddhist nuns, books by long-dead philosophers and poets. I learn that I am not my thoughts, I am just the person who hears them. I discover that I do not need to know, I just need to let go. I float around repeating these phrases and affirmations as if my life depends on them.

It does.

I realise how very, very mentally unwell I have been for the last three years; how close I came to setting fire to everything. I reflect on the power and tenacity of mental illness. Even when you think you know it intimately, when you believe you have learned all its most cunning and conniving ways, you can never know it fully – and perhaps that is for the best. I think about the menopause, and how at first I believed it had made everything worse. But now I start to wonder if actually, perimenopause might have been the very thing that woke me up and allowed me to start getting *better*.

I read about Carl Jung, and how he saw ageing as an awakening and believed that there were no accidents in life. It chimes with me, not least because the pretentious prat in me likes the idea of sitting and reading about Jungian psychology. But mostly I like the notion because it makes me think about the timing of the diagnosis of my atrial fibrillation, just a week after the coil was put inside me. I think how scared and stressed I was back at the beginning of the year, how utterly depleted I had been by all my previous experiences of trying to get progesterone into my body. I think about how, if the coil hadn't worked, the next step would have been a hysterectomy. I think about how the diagnosis of A-Fib forced me to take my mental and physical health seriously, how it was actually the moment when I started to turn a corner. It was a wake-up call. A plea from my heart to take precious care of it.

I lose myself in the Spirituality and Self-Help section of Foyles, a place that a previous version of me might have laughed at – or worse, sneered at. But that version of me spent her time in the Soho bars in the streets surrounding Foyles, drinking and drugging her soul into a state of mute misery. Who am I to argue with the words of Brené Brown, Louise Hay, Roger Teel or Carl Jung?

19

Woo-hoo

Snapshot from my iPhone Notes App, May 2023

< Notes   ↑   ⋯

PLEEEEEASE CAN I GET A PHONE I WILL CLEAN MY BEDROOM AND
YOUR BEDROOM AND MAKE YOU DINNER
From Edie

☰   📷   Ⓐ   ✎

Edith calls to check in on me.

'How are you getting on with the coil, darling?' she says.

'Well, we seem to be getting on fine so far,' I say, truthfully. There have been one or two tearful days, but I have spent them doing CrossFit and chanting Louise Hay's affirmations, which

I think has helped. 'I'm hoping we can be friends. Me and the coil. Me and *you*, Edith.'

'Darling, now I've seen inside your vagina, I promise you we are the best of friends.'

We talk a bit more, as friends do. I tell her about my quest to read all of the self-help books. Edith tells me about a book she read when her husband left her for his secretary.

'Such a cliché,' she sighs, 'but in truth the best thing that could have happened to me. Anyway, the book changed my life. I re-read it twice a year, when I'm not fitting coils into people's wombs.'

The book – *Women Who Run with the Wolves* – is by a writer called Clarissa Pinkola Estés. The sight of it causes my husband to take an audibly deep breath when I climb into bed with it that night, but I am here for it. The book, not the deep breathing.

Pinkola Estés writes about how culture forces women to water themselves down until they are mere holograms of themselves. I gasp at her prose, at her description of a woman 'harassed by the petty demands of her psyche which exhort her to comply with whatever anyone wishes. Compliance causes a shocking realisation that must be registered by all women. That is, to be ourselves causes us to exiled by many others, and yet to comply with what others want causes us to be exiled from ourselves.'

I think about all the people pleasing I have done, to the detriment of my own happiness. All the times I have put other people's needs above my own. I think of all the moments I have said yes to things when I really meant no, and all the effort I have spent contorting my body into impossible shapes to make everybody else comfortable, as if I were a chaise longue and not a human who occasionally needs to lie flat herself. I think about the fear I have of being in trouble, fear I carry in my heart like a

298

four-year-old. But I am not four. I am a forty-two-year-old, and it is time I started treating myself like one. I love this Clarissa chick. She is my queen.

'When she is starved,' writes Pinkola Estés, 'a woman will take any substitutes offered, including those that ... do absolutely nothing for her, as well as destructive and life-threatening ones that hideously waste her time and talents or expose her life to physical danger. It is a famine of the soul that makes a woman choose things that will cause her to dance madly out of control – then too, too near the executioner's door.'

I think about getting this tattooed down my arm, but abandon my plans when I realise that I might run out of skin. But the words feel etched on my heart in such a way that I start to feel a sort of rage. A rage with myself, for being a willing participant in my own degradation. This didn't just happen to me – I allowed it to. I invited it in. I went along with all the rhetoric that told me I had to be smaller, sexier, less shrill. I saw it not as a threat to my wellbeing, but a condition of it. Now, as I read Pinkola Estés, I feel my brain coming back to life.

'Sometimes it is difficult for us to realise when we are losing our instincts, for it is an insidious process that does not occur all in one day, but rather over a long period of time.'

Has Clarissa Pinkola Estés been observing my life for the last three years?

'Too, the loss or deadening of instinct is often entirely supported by the surrounding culture, and sometimes even by other women who endure the loss of instinct as a way of achieving belonging in a culture that keeps no nourishing habitat for the natural woman.'

Pinkola Estés points to how ancient women would 'often set a sacred place aside' to come together and that 'traditionally, it is said to have been set aside during women's menses, for [this is] a time that woman lives much closer to self-knowing than usual; the membrane between the unconscious and conscious minds thins considerably.'

She talks about the effects of removing these sacred spaces for women from society. 'My experience in analysing women leads me to believe that much of modern women's premenstrual crankiness is not just a physical syndrome but is equally attributable to her being thwarted in her need to take enough time away to revivify and renew herself. I always laugh when I hear someone quoting early anthropologists who claimed that menstruating women of various tribes were considered "unclean" and forced to leave the village until they were "over it". All women know that even if there were such a forced ritual exile, every single woman, to a woman, would, when her time came, leave the village hanging her head mournfully, at least till she was out of sight, and then suddenly break into a jig down the path, cackling all the way.'

The truth of this lands in the centre of my chest with a thud. It occurs to me that sometimes, simply existing as a woman is enough to make you ill. But as I lie there, contemplating the words of Clarissa Pinkola Estés, I begin to question my own negativity regarding the menopause. Instead of being a miserable experience that ruins women and casts them on to the rubbish heap, could it be that the whole process is actually an opportunity? Could it be that there is a witchy magic to it? I have railed against my own early menopause because it seemed to me that it swept in and took away all the things I had worked so bloody hard to build since I was a teenager: self-esteem, confidence, the ability to juggle a career and a family and all the other things I was told I could – *should* – have. But reading *Women Who Run with the Wolves,* I am struck by the thought that all the emotional things brought up by the menopause could actually be our bodies and our souls highlighting the issues we need to deal with if we want the second half of our lives to be truly worthwhile. Not worthwhile in the way society says. Worthwhile in the way *we* want.

That overwhelming imposter syndrome that's got really bad in the last three years?

That's got to go.

That ridiculous people-pleasing that has become so very pronounced recently?

That's got to go.

The endless hypervigilance to ensure nobody thinks I am bad?

That's got to go.

The giving away of my power in the hope that it makes other people's lives easier?

That's got to go.

The believing that I am a product with a sell-by date, rather than a human?

That's got to go.

It's all got to go.

It all has to change.

From now on, I stop saying no to myself.

From now on, I only say yes to my soul.

And anyone who thinks I'm behaving like a mad woman?

Well, obviously, they've got to go, too.

20

Naked

Snapshot from my iPhone's Notes App, July 2023

OK MUM, WHAT ABOUT A DOG INSTEAD OF A PHONE?
From Edie

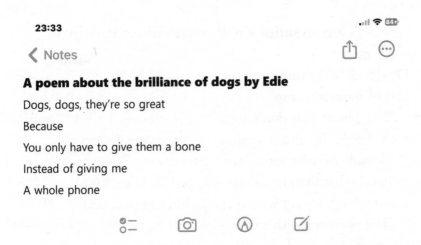

For my forty-third birthday, I treat myself to a . . . well, a retreat.

To give you some idea of how momentous this is: for my twenty-fourth birthday, a friend gave me a silver straw through which to snort cocaine (no idea what happened to it); I once had a birthday party that went on for so long – and so loudly – that I was later evicted after the local neighbourhood watch banded together to complain to the landlady (fair enough); I spent my thirtieth doing lines of coke off a car bonnet, having lost my keys during an all-day bender at a pub (not my finest moment).

A retreat is to a woman in her forties what a week in Ayia Napa is to one in her early twenties: a sort of rite of passage, I suppose. Some people go to retreats in Bali or Ibiza or Greece, where they stay silent for days on end and learn to stand on their heads. I choose one in Haywards Heath, because I only have a weekend and, honestly, I've never much liked flying (or the idea of standing on my head in silence). It is a two-day course for women, called 'Naked', and I think it is a tribute to how much I have grown that this doesn't leave me laughing/rolling my eyes/both.

Conversations with my mother: Part five

Obviously, my mum assumes it means I have signed up to some sort of naturist camp.

'No, Mum, you don't have to get *actually* naked,' I explain with a sigh. 'It's more about getting *emotionally* naked.'

'Sounds horrific either way.' She snorts. 'Are you sure you'd rather do that than let us take you out for cake? Honestly, I don't know what's wrong with a good old-fashioned party.'

'The problem with a good old-fashioned party,' I say, 'is that I no longer *like* good old-fashioned parties. God, it's such a relief to actually say that out loud. I've been trying to convince myself for the whole of my sobriety that I will one day enjoy going out in the evening again, and you know what? I'm calling it and saying: "Nope, not for me, never been for me, actually." In fact, maybe the pressure to go to good old-fashioned parties was *part* of the reason I ended up drinking so much, because deep down in secret, I'm horrifically shy and anxious about meeting new people – AND THAT'S OK!'

'Woo-hoo, Happy Birthday to you! Just one thing, though, Bryony. Shy people don't tend to spend their weekends with strangers on retreats called "Naked". Are you *sure* that's what you want to do?'

'I am sure, Mum,' I say. 'After all, isn't "taking herself seriously" the greatest gift a woman can give to herself?'

'Well, now, there's taking yourself seriously and then there's sitting in a field talking about your feelings.'

'It's not in a field! It's in a hall!'

'If that's how you want to spend your birthday, I'm terrifically proud of you. I'm sure it will be very interesting, and I will look forward to hearing how it goes. Now, I must get on. I've got to go and start taking *myself* seriously, so that by the time *my* birthday rolls around, I can actually bear to admit how old I am. That's quite enough emotional nudity for me, I think!'

Naked takes place in a small church hall somewhere off the Lewes Road. It is all about embracing the divine feminine, which is a phrase I've heard in some of the many self-help books I've been reading, but one that I'm still not quite sure I understand. Is it something to do with masturbation? I hope not. Which reminds me: all that sexual shame around desire and fantasy and orgasms?

Eventually, that's gotta go.

There are eight of us, including a highly qualified therapist who will facilitate the weekend. We sit on the floor of the hall, very much clothed, very much not encouraged to masturbate, surrounded by candles, yoga bolsters and vases full of freshly picked wild flowers. It's not my place to tell you about the other women on the course, but what I will say – and I'm sure they won't mind me saying it – is that while our reasons for being there are varied, we all also have one thing in common: we have all reached the point of giving up on ourselves. We've reached the point, through divorce or menopause or violence or addiction, or whatever else it is that has woken up the Still Small Voice, and we have decided we can no longer do this. We can no longer abandon our wants and our needs and our desires on a daily basis in order to please a society that has no interest whatsoever in pleasing *us*.

We are saying no to expectations.

And yes to ourselves.

One by one, the therapist invites us to step into the circle and get emotionally naked. To let everything out without fear of being judged. She asks us what it is we want to face, to deal with, and then, over the course of an hour and a half, she helps us face that thing, with the support of the other women. Then we go through a series of somatic exercises, such as shaking our bodies and screaming at the tops of our lungs, to help us release whatever it is we have been holding on to all these years.

And as we stand there, gyrating our hips around in a church hall, shaking our arms wildly in the air and screaming all sorts of expletives into the room, I think I must look completely mad. Objectively, I have never actually looked madder. But something dawns on me, as I watch the other women holler and howl, and it is this: I am not mad. I have never been mad. The OCD, the alcoholism, the alopecia, the eating disorders, the depression, the endless fucking anxiety . . . they were all completely appropriate. They were my brain trying to show me what was wrong with my life. They were a complex response to a simple truth: that I have never accepted myself as I am.

My mental illnesses were actually healthy brain responses to living in a world that only wanted me *good*. A world that wanted me small, compliant, biddable; that wanted me not to take up too much space that might be better used by someone else, someone male. A world that wanted me to look hot, be quiet, smile sweetly, act nice, make money, have kids, not complain. A world that wanted me to be the kind of woman that doesn't allow for being human.

Jareth, the Stay Puft Marshmallow Man, and all of the rest of them . . . they weren't enemies, trying to bring me down.

My brain created them, to try and help me cope.

My clever, clever brain. My super-strong soul.

I am not mad.

I am *fucking amazing*.

Conversations with my mother: Part six

'Darling, how was the Nude weekend?'

'It was great. Actually, I think you'd have got a lot from it. Maybe one day you can treat yourself to a Nude weekend.'

'I don't think so, Bryony! Now, I still need to see you to celebrate your birthday. When can we make this happen?'

'So, I was thinking on Saturday? The woman from the Nude weekend has set us all some homework, and I was hoping you'd come and do it with me.'

'I was thinking more that you could all come round for lunch or something.'

'Mum, I promise this will be more special. And I promise you it doesn't involve getting nude. Well, not physically, anyway.'

'OK, have it your way.'

Today, we are letting go of the things that no longer serve us.

I have found two smooth, brown rocks, and got myself some Sharpie pens, as the woman from Naked suggested. The plan is to write on these rocks the thing we want to release. The thing that has been holding us back from dazzling in our full light.

Then we are to go to a body of water, and throw the rocks in.

When I explain this to my mother, she tells me there isn't enough space on the rock. 'I'm going to need more of a paving stone to write down all the flaws I want to let go of,' she says, holding the Sharpie aloft. 'Perhaps even an entire cement wall.'

'I wish you'd be kinder to yourself,' I say.

'I wish I would be, too. OK, let's get on with this ridiculous ritual, and then maybe you'll let us all have some goddamn birthday cake.'

We sit quietly at the kitchen table with our thoughts. I think of all the stones I could scrawl on, of the vast, rocky beach out there that could be filled with parts of me I don't like. Shame. Intrusive thoughts. Crow's feet. The heaviness of my tits. My constant need to get from A to Z without first going through B, C, D, and so on. The fact I still miss smoking. And chorizo. My tendency to snap when my husband doesn't do something exactly the way I want him to. My alcoholism. The men I should have told to fuck off, but instead ended up saying 'I love you' to, because what's that about? My lack of style. My inability to reply to texts. The fact I still don't really like going out at night, and that I still look at my phone while I'm eating. The fact I don't know how to do a proper roast. That I'm selfish. That I don't think about other people enough.

There are so many rocks that have weighed me down and caused me pain. I would need to rent an entire HGV to be able to take all my rocks to the sea. Then I'd put my back out throwing them in.

What if I were to sit down with those rocks, and instead of frantically trying to throw them away, I just left them as they were? What if I tried to see the bigger picture, of all the rocks together, and how they actually make up something kind of beautiful? Messy and uncomfortable but beautiful all the same. What if I were to realise that a vast, rocky beach is just as important as a white, sandy one?

'I think I know what I want to get rid of,' announces my mother, proudly.

I scribble on my stone. Then I put it in my pocket, and enjoy the sensation of it weighing me down one last time.

I take her to the banks of the Thames, near our home in south London. We sit on a bench overlooking the murky brown water.

There is a chill in the air, despite it being July. The sky is overcast, and the tide is quite far out, revealing the muddy bed of the river and all the rubbish that lies there.

'Well, isn't this lovely?' says my mum, looking at the e-bike someone has thrown over the wall and into the silt. 'I hope my throw is good enough to get my rock into the water.'

'The tide will come in and wash it away, wherever it lands,' I say. 'Did you know a whale was found dead under Battersea Bridge once? If the Thames can take away a whole minke whale, it can take away the two stones that are holding us back.'

'Poor whale,' says my mum. 'Poor *us*, reduced to drawing on rocks to celebrate your birthday.'

'No more negativity, Mum!' I smile at her. 'Now, are you ready to throw away your stone?'

'I sure am!' She gets it out of her pocket and clears her throat. 'I'm letting go of the need to please people who behave like arseholes. I couldn't fit all of that on the stone, though, so I've just written "arseholes".' She waves the rock in a jolly manner, stands up, and throws it towards the river.

I look at the small, smooth rock in my hand, and I kiss it. I take a deep breath, hold it close to me one last time. Then, with all the force I have in my body, I hurl it into the air. I watch as it rises and rises into the gloomy sky, spinning as it goes. Then it begins to fall, down, down, down, hitting the water with a splash that feels almost shocking to me.

The rock is quickly swallowed, carried off to goodness knows where.

I feel only a little bit sad.

Goodbye, Jareth.

Hello, me.

Acknowledgments

My endless gratitude goes to my agent Nelle Andrew, who has believed in me even – and especially – when I haven't been able to believe in myself. A huge thanks to everyone at Headline for making me the mad woman and author I am today: Yvonne Jacob, Raiyah Butt, Louise Swannell, Lucy Howkins, Tina Paul, Mari Evans, as well as Tara O'Sullivan and everyone who has worked on the six (!) books that Headline have published.

Thank you to Becca Barr for raising me up, and to Emma Lucy and Becky Knowles for encouraging me to dazzle. Thank you Holly Beck, Laura Cole, Becca Priestley, Martha Freud and Emma Campbell for being in my life. I couldn't have done any of this without the help of Tertius Richardson and Jess Griffiths. Big shout out to the community at Shapesmiths for your infectious energy and encouragement. To Kate Whale, Dean Piper, Rick Parcell, Anthony Richmond and all the team at BodyCamp, thank you for bringing me back to the light after some very dark days indeed. I am endlessly grateful to Jenny Masterman for her kindness in letting me stay at her Spanish sanctuary, where a lot of this book was written. Gracias!

Thanks Mum and Dad, Naomi and Rufus for EV-ERY-THING. And to Harry and Edie. I love our little team, always and forever.

Further resources

If you think you need help, the following organisations provide great support for people affected by issues covered in this book:

MIND
www.mind.org.uk
0300 123 3393 or info@mind.org.uk

Beat
www.beateatingdisorders.org.uk
080 801 0677 or help@beateatingdisorders.org.uk

The Menopause Charity
www.menopausecharity.org
Go to their website for resources on menopause and mental health.

CALM (Campaign Against Living Miserably)
www.thecalmzone.net
0800 58 58 58 or use their anonymous write-in service on their website.

Mental Health Mates
www.mentalhealthmates.co.uk
Go to their website for information on how to get involved.

Papyrus
www.papyrus-uk.org
0800 068 41 41, text 07860 039 967 or pat@papyrus-uk.org

OCD UK
www.ocduk.org
01332 588112 or support@ocduk.org